Dr. Hip's Natural Food & Unnatural Acts

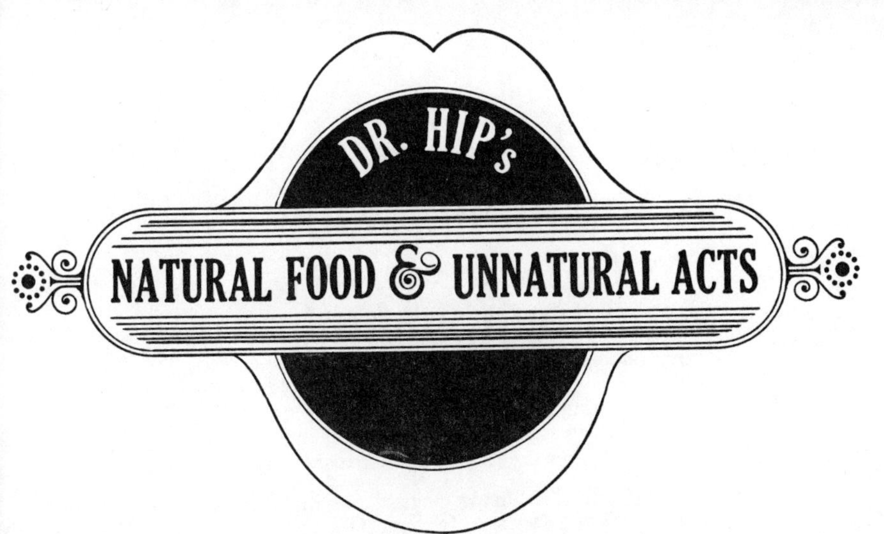

Eugene Schoenfeld, M.D.

DELACORTE PRESS • SEYMOUR LAWRENCE

Manufactured in the United States of America
Designed by Jerry Tillett
First printing

Portions of "The Granola Papers" appeared in the January 4, 1973, *Rolling Stone*.

"How to Produce A ~~Rock Concert~~ Disaster" is published courtesy of Straight Arrow Publications. It was one of the personal accounts used for *Rolling Stone*'s prizewinning story of the Altamont Rock Concert.

Library of Congress Cataloging in Publication Data

Schoenfeld, Eugene, 1935–
Dr. Hip's natural food & unnatural acts.

Includes bibliographies.
1. Questions and answers—Hygiene, Sexual.
2. Questions and answers—Narcotics. 3. Medicine—Miscellanea. I. Title.
RA788.S36 613.9'5 74-5303

ISBN: 0-440-03288-1

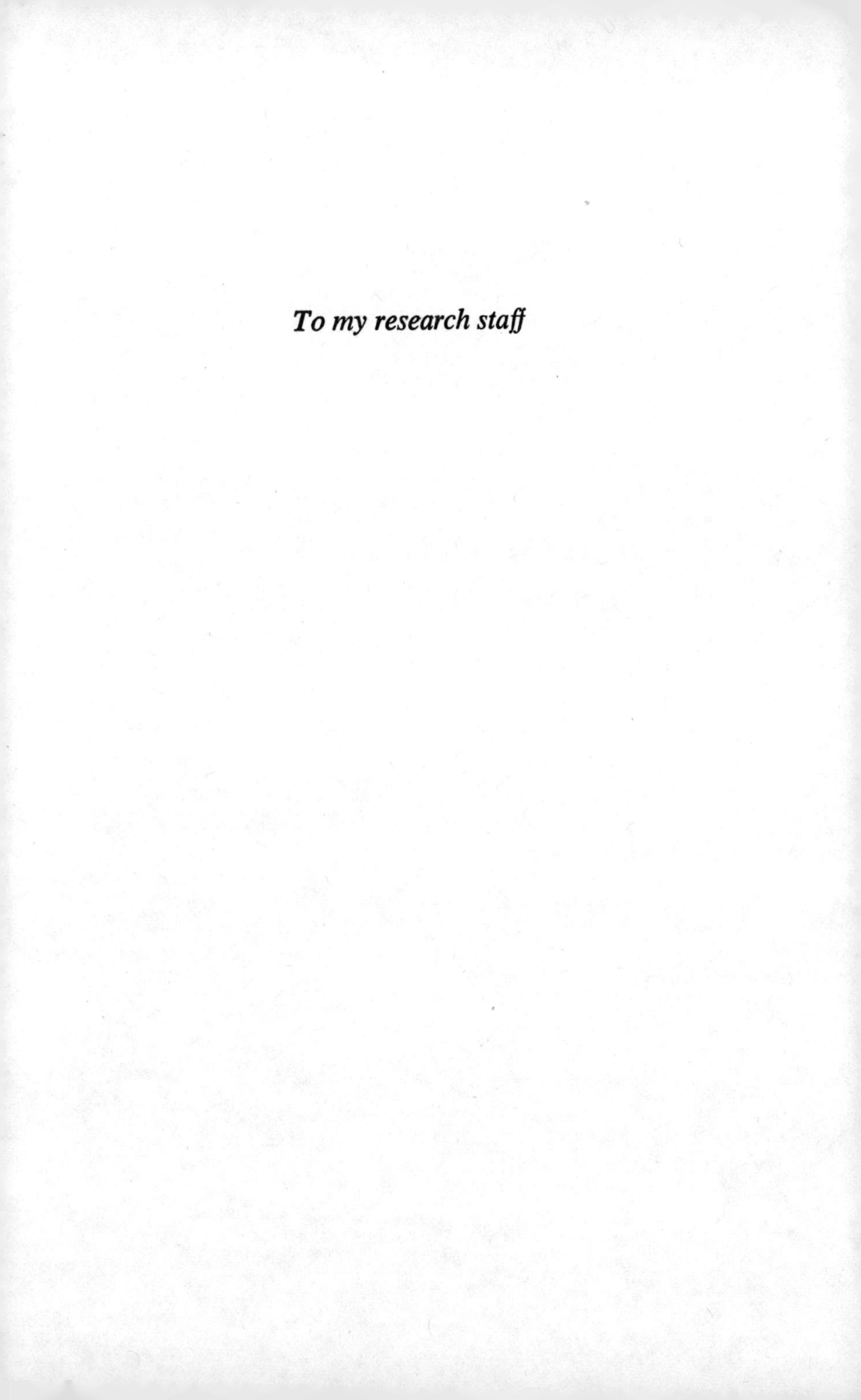

To my research staff

Contents

Introduction

Writing a weekly newspaper column is probably like making it with an insatiable gorilla. The minute you're finished, you've got to start all over again.

JUDITH WESTON,
former weekly columnist

During a summer spent at the Albert Schweitzer Hospital in Gabon, I roomed with a three-year-old gorilla named Peter. The Swiss nurse who'd cared for him previously was returning home after four years in Africa. I happily volunteered to look after Peter and his cage was moved to my room.

Peter was brought to the hospital by African hunters who'd killed his mother. He was Dr. Schweitzer's special pet and the old man (he was 85 then) gave me careful instructions about raising young gorillas. Since Peter had lived among people since infancy, he was very much like a furry, incredibly strong and mischievous child.

Each morning I'd dress him in a blue denim harness and he'd accompany me on my rounds or sit by a palm tree learning tricks like thumping his chest or smashing lengths of bamboo into splinters.

Peter unattended indoors meant the end of habitation as I knew it. He stayed in the wooden pen if I had to leave him in our room alone or when we slept. He was afraid of the dark and whimpered like a baby at night unless someone remained with him or I lit a kerosene lamp. The nurses called him "Peterli," little Peter. Sometimes I called him other names.

By summer's end Peter was stronger than most adult humans. I had to return to medical school in the fall and Peter couldn't have made it in the jungle alone. Dr. Schweitzer's daughter Rhena flew to Denmark with Peter and gave him to the Copenhagen zoo where I used to visit him every year or so. My little friend grew into a gigantic creature who liked tearing off his keeper's clothes. Before he developed that habit, I was allowed inside the cage, which sometimes startled people on the other side of the bars and glass.

Naturally, I was interested in Ms. Weston's reference to gorillas and columns. Gorillaphiles who've spent months and years living out-of-doors amongst ADULT gorillas report their sexual prowess is greatly overrated. A few humps, a few grunts, and it's all over. But Judith Weston's analogy to writing a newspaper column has the smell of truth about it. And apropos of nothing except gorillas, I've heard there's a beastly erotic scene censored from most versions of *King Kong*. When the great brute carries Fay Wray in his hands for the first time, he's said to afterward sniff one of his fingers.

From March 24, 1967, until July 15, 1973, I wrote my Hip Pocrates medical column each week except for a month during the spring of 1970 while touring riot-torn college campuses. The column began in the *Berkeley Barb*, received its name from *Barb* editor Max Scherr, and soon was carried by many other underground publications. Later, Hip Pocrates appeared also in a dozen more-or-less straight newspapers including the San Francisco *Chronicle*, Chicago *Sun-Times*, San Antonio *Express*, Philadelphia *News* and Minneapolis *Star-Tribune*.

I started the column because the need for factual public information on taboo subjects like sex and drugs was evident and I welcomed the opportunity to write. My first two columns came from questions friends or patients personally asked me. After that I used only letters received by mail and they were a continual source of information, provocation, amusement, amazement, joy and sorrow.

Sometimes I used no questions, writing instead about events I observed or issues which seemed important or interesting. Usually those columns were somehow related to medicine too. There were columns on the first and bloodiest People's Park demonstration, the Kent State killings, a visit to the Indians occupying Alcatraz Island, the wretched conditions in most American nursing homes, police smashing ambulances in the Washington, D.C., May Day demonstrations against the Vietnam War. While I valued reaching millions of newspaper readers through the straight press, the limitations imposed were soon evident. Many columns weren't printed in the dailies. In March 1972 I warned that government agents often deviously obtained confidential medical information. The dailies refused to print it.

My answers to medical questions often differed from the official American Medical Association party line, especially about sex and drugs. But I backed my statements with evidence and tried to make clear which areas remained controversial. The straight press published almost all the drug information.

A few daily newspapers were willing to print frank descriptions about sex—giving and getting head, for example, if terms like cunnilingus and fellatio were used. "Balling" was okay with the San Francisco *Chronicle* but "fucking" wasn't.

Though most of our states have laws providing severe legal penalties for most sexual acts, even between consenting adults, these laws are rarely enforced. A Los Angeles case involving oral sex was thrown out of court by the presiding judge recently on the obvious ground that the state has no business peeking into people's bedrooms. The Attorney General of California, though, said the judge's ruling applies only to Los Angeles. Theoretically, if your head should bob across the Los Angeles County line to Orange County, it's one to fourteen years in prison. But these laws are hardly ever invoked except to bust the cast or producers of erotic films or live stage shows.

The other major topic covered in my columns involved drugs. Drugs! The Red-baiting, Red-hunting hysteria of McCarthyism in the 1950's was replaced by the menace of mind-altering drugs. Like any movement involving fad elements, there were (and are) people involved for all the wrong reasons. Those of us who worked with students or in drug treatment clinics soon observed and treated many casualties of the drug revolution.

Documented cases of deaths associated with drugs like LSD certainly did occur. One of my friends was on duty at Berkeley's student health service when police carried in the body of a girl who looked in a mirror while tripping and saw reflected a grotesque mask (remember that one? usually it's one half the face). Unlike most people who see the horrors in a mirror, this girl ran through her apartment, dived out a window and fell four floors, landing on her face.

We all know about drug-associated deaths (let's forget for the moment the most destructive drug by far—alcohol). Jimi Hendrix, Janis Joplin, Jim Morrison, Gram Parsons are some. We know about people who don't do anything much except drugs—the ones, we're told falsely, who are amotivational *because* of drugs. Yes, we know the harm people can cause themselves. And many of us also know the beneficial uses of drugs, including pleasure.

"Drug experts" usually ignore the way personal experiences and concepts of individual freedom influence their judgments of drug use and "abuse." Drug abuse often means "drug use I don't like."

I've always tried to be very clear about my own views of drug use. The government has no right to interfere with private behavior involving "victimless crimes" of any type. Imprisoning people for possession or use of drugs is more catastrophic to a society than any effect of drugs. As a service to the public, the government ought to certify their chemical purity, indicate potential uses, dangers and which are best under medical supervision. A person untrained in medicine who self-prescribes dangerous drugs like antibiotics is, in my opinion, a fool. But should governments legislate against foolishness?

Basically that's where I am on the drug issue. Dismantle the Gestapo-like army of narcs and eliminate drug laws as we know them. The first laws dealing with narcotics in the United States were passed in 1914—the Harrison Narcotic Act. We had a lot of narcotic addicts before the Harrison Narcotic Act was put into law—that was the reason given for its enactment. *Today the United States has exactly the same proportion of narcotic addicts.* But we've also had hundreds of thousands of drug prisoners, brutal armed psychopaths with badges terrorizing victims of fascist no-knock laws, and a president who could divert attention from the most corrupt administration in U.S. history by saying, "Drug abuse is public enemy number one."

I hardly ever referred to my drug experiences. Anyone known to the public soon learns there are people who will emulate behavior because of positive identification. Or trust. Once someone asked me if LSD impaired memory. My answer was that I couldn't remember reading any such reports. My belief is that mature people ought to have the opportunity to try psychedelic drugs if they wish to, in conditions most conducive to a good experience.

LSD is an extraordinarily powerful psychedelic. But LSD is but the crude prototype of beneficial chemicals which might be developed in a free civilization.

At first many people thought, "By God, everyone should take LSD!" Maybe you met some along the way, proselytizing for psychedelics the same way they ranted against the very same drugs later. True believers bring powerful energies to whatever new cause they may support. But they remain true believers. Not long ago a member of the staff of Berkeley's student psychiatric service said something like "Everyone should try marijuana." Everyone? Bullshit. If there is something, some food, some drug, some belief even, that benefits *everyone*, I'd like to know it. That same psychiatrist today is a rabid foe of marijuana use, claiming he can recognize users by their "puppet-like" walk. How's your gait, buddy?

As more drug information became generally available I devoted less space to the topic in my column. Nothing new was happening with drugs and I didn't like going over old territory. More attention was paid to a broader range of medical subjects including nutrition. We had a lot of fun around the office when granola was found no more nutritious than commercial dry cereals.

Though I'd considered stopping the column several times, the decision came easily after a telephone conversation with an editor of a large newspaper.

"But Doctor," he said, "we're *buying* a question-answer column on sex and drugs." Not mine, I thought, and stopped the column.

This book is mostly based on my medical columns, uncensored and rearranged by chapters. The answers to many letters came from personal experiences and that's why I've included articles like the Altamont Rock Concert/Disaster, The Granola Papers and a freakish Alternative Media Conference.

While much of the information in this book comes from my own experience, I have relied heavily on the consultants listed below. My "research staff" of friends and acquaintances have made extraordinary contributions, often in my kitchen as I opened the day's mail, as well as other places.

One of the most invaluable things I've learned is that a secretary can be the most important member of a work team, functioning as memory, guide and provocateur. Mine have usually been with me part-time or on a temporary basis, like Sandra McLanahan who took a year's leave from medical school. Thanks are due to Jacki Ruby, Jeanne Cluff-Cochran, Barbara Quinn, Honor Thompson, Linda Goorland, Judi Sawyer, Jeanne Lance, Sandra McLanahan, Joanne Kyger (this talented poetess was kind enough to help a neighbor), Sally Moses, Rona Elliot, Andrea Belsky and Pauline Stamberger.

When Hip Pocrates first began I wondered if there would

ever be an end to new questions. There seems no possibility that that will occur in the foreseeable future, a good sign I think. For we may expect human evolution to continue only so long as questions outnumber answers.

EUGENE SCHOENFELD, M.D.
Stinson Beach, California

List of Consultants

William Alexander, M.D.	Psychiatry
Sterling Bunnell, M.D.	Psychiatry
Vasilios Choulos	Law
Consumers Cooperative Nutritionists	Nutrition
John Davis, M.D.	Endocrinology
John Doss, M.D.	Pediatrics
Joel Fort, M.D.	Psychiatry
B. G. Gross, M.D.	Dermatology
James M. Harris, D.V.M.	Veterinary Medicine
G. Legman	Oragenitalism
Sheldon Margen, M.D.	Nutrition
William Robbins, D.D.S.	Dentistry
Gil Roberts, M.D.	Family Medicine
Fred Rohe	Nutrition
Morris Schambelan, M.D.	Internal Medicine
Martin Schneider	Medical Oddities
Frank Schoenfeld, M.D.	Psychiatry
Adolph Segal, M.D.	Orthopedics
Alexander Shulgin, Ph.D.	Biochemistry
Margo St. James	Sexology
Michael Stepanian	Law

1

Natural Food and Unnatural Acts

Nutrition

Nutrition is still a dark, mysterious subject in the health sciences so it is not surprising most people know little about maintaining and improving their health through proper diet. When I was a medical student nutrition was virtually ignored except for the vitamins, biochemical processes and diets for specific medical diseases. Small wonder then so many fad diets, some dangerous, flourish in the counterculture.

Fortunately, the human organism can adapt to a great variety of diets, ranging from all meat to no meat, even including some of the less extreme macrobiotic regimes. There is no doubt certain diets can affect one's health and mind adversely through starvation. But there's little or no scientific proof for the curative potential of nutrition. Like astrology, it deserves a complete scientific investigation to enable people either to stop wasting their time, money (and bodies) or to benefit from new knowledge.

I view the boom in "organic" or natural foods as a very healthy trend, though too often carried to unnatural extremes. Vegetarianism removes the need to kill animals for food. But when we are told vegetarians are not aggressive, the mind leaps to notable exceptions like Adolf Hitler and Charles Manson. Some food faddists use the rationalization that Hitler's actions can be blamed on his fondness for sugary confections, a belief which can only be explained by low blood sugar in the faddists holding these deranged opinions.

To get an idea of what frightens many about prepackaged, long-shelf-life foods, take a look at the ingredients of "nondairy creamers." Are they really less harmful than real cream? Next time you cut into a piece of prime U.S. beef, consider that Sweden will continue banning the importation of U.S. cattle so long as hormones like diethylstilbestrol are injected in order to increase the animal's weight. Those little dessert tins of butterscotch and chocolate pudding look and even taste delicious, but what are those strange chemicals listed on the side of the can contributing to the life-span of the average American?

I recently received a letter in which the writer related a new way of getting high. He took a handful of raisins, ate them, then took another handful, put them in his cheek and slowly chewed, extracting and swallowing the juice. He stated this altered time sense, produced visions and aroused his sexual appetite.

That same morning as I sat in my kitchen research laboratory, mouth full of raisins, I reflected upon the seemingly never-ending search for mind-altering experiences, a universal human interest which cannot be quelled by threats of prison terms, social and economic reprisals or, at times, even accurate information about real dangers.

As I expected, there was no noticeable alteration in my consciousness. One of my appetites was sated but it was only that for sweets.

Later I received a letter that said, "Maybe what's making those raisin eaters high is the sulfur dioxide with which fruits are likewise treated."

And it was true I had been eating so-called organic raisins. Although I am not a food faddist I think, given a choice, I always opt for food that does not have chemicals intentionally added.

Chemical additives aside, the relationship between drugs, food and the mind is a most interesting one, an area in its early stages of exploration—at least in the West.

Are vitamins drugs, for example? The Food and Drug Administration wants the authority to regulate in this area. Some psychiatrists believe megavitamin therapy is useful in treating certain psychoses. Many reports indicate niacin in quantities of 500 mgm or larger will abort an LSD trip.

And finally there *is* definite proof of the mind-altering potential of raisins.

Dear Dr. Schoenfeld:

You can *get high on raisins.*

Enclosed is a raisin winemaking kit for you. It makes two gallons, and the wine tastes delicious.

We have been selling raisin winemaking kits for over a year now. Anyone who would like one can order them from us for $2.00 each.

We hope you have fun with it.

California Raisin Advisory Board
P.O. Box 5335
Fresno, California 93755

Asparagus Season

Dear Dr. Schoenfeld:

Well, here it is asparagus season. After I eat asparagus, my urine acquires a very strong odor. My girlfriend notices that she experiences the same thing. Is this unusual?

Do you know what it is that causes the strong smell? Does your lab assistant notice it too?

ANSWER: One out of every seven people has an enzyme variation causing a peculiarly pungent odor to the urine after asparagus is eaten. These individuals undoubtedly share other genetic characteristics as well but they haven't yet been identified.

My laboratory assistant has noticed this phenomenon all right but not in herself.

Chinese Restaurant Syndrome

Dear Dr Schoenfeld:

Whenever I eat in a Chinese restaurant the upper part of my body feels numb, I feel weak all over and my heart seems to pound.

What could be wrong?

ANSWER: Chinese Restaurant Syndrome came to public attention with the publication of a letter in the *New England Journal of Medicine* from Dr. Robert Ho Man Kwok. He noted the symptoms you mention when dining in Chinese restaurants but not when eating home-cooked Chinese food.

Even before Dr. Kwok's letter appeared, a Yale gastroenterologist had found a connection between Chinese food and headaches in some individuals. Dr. Martin Gordon and seven brave volunteers (all of whom had previously been victims of Chinese Restaurant Syndrome) ate in a Chinese restaurant in New Haven, Connecticut.

Halfway through the meal they noticed headaches, numbness of the face, palpitation of the heart, sweating, clenched jaws and flushed faces.

The culprit seems to be monosodium glutamate (MSG) which is generally used in such delicacies as won ton soup. Most people are not sensitive to this seasoning but those who are suffer from the dread Chinese Restaurant Syndrome.

Don't worry too much about it. One or two hours after the symptoms begin they disappear and you'll be hungry again.

Roman Gorgy

Dear Dr. Schoenfeld:

For the past two years my husband, 29 years old, has been indulging in a bad practice—self-induced regurgitation. In other words, he eats all he wants, then sticks his fingers down his throat and vomits it all up.

He does this every day, always at least three times, sometimes four times, every day. This has been going on for two years now. This is the way he controls his weight. I have tried to tell him that once a day and I wouldn't mind, but 3 or 4 times a day makes me very upset. Also, I wonder if he could damage his throat or stomach in any way.

Every day, starting about 1:00 p.m. he starts eating. First it's a meat pattie and egg or cottage cheese for breakfast and after that nothing stays in his stomach. A typical sam-

ple of his daily gluttony: ½ lb. peanuts, a large bag of potato chips, 1 dozen donuts, 6 candy bars, 1 large bowl of popcorn, 3 or 4 bottles of soft drinks (dietetic, of course), ½ gallon of ice cream, 10 or 12 chocolate candies, a full meal (if we go out and eat). Every day without fail he eats 1 large bowl of popcorn, and ½ gallon of ice cream and usually peanuts, potato chips or both. This goes on until about 1:00 a.m. Then he vomits for the last time about 12:30 a.m., takes his vitamins and goes to bed. Then it starts all over again the next day.

He also has been out of work for over a year, and has a frightening temper. This I can put up with but the vomiting is terrible. I have begged, pleaded, threatened and ignored the problem. I even sent him to a psychiatrist but the psychiatrist said it was OK to do it. From time to time he makes promises that he will quit but he never does. No one knows about it but me.

P.S. I have stopped making dinners at night such as a good meat dish, vegetables, etc., as he just throws it up and it's all wasted. Our food bill for two runs about $50 a week and his parents pay for it. So that's another problem. They don't know about his problem but wonder why he stays so thin. Just lately he is starting to have a drink in the evening once in a while. He never drank except if we went out. His family places great importance on eating, and they are all overweight. I know this is why he is that way but I don't know how to stop him.

ANSWER: Not long ago, I met a girl who told me she and her roommate practiced the same unusual method of weight control. They were living in Paris at the time and really dug the food. But they kept gaining weight. Instead of throwing up their hands, they sacrificed their meals.

Fasting is an acceptable way to lose weight under a physician's supervision but the methods described here add the risk of upsetting the body's chemical balance through loss of gastric fluids. Severe retching can also cause rupturing of the stomach with fatal results.

Maybe we *are* returning to the days of ancient Rome. Peel me a (union) grape, someone.

DDT and Mother's Milk

Dear Dr. Schoenfeld:

The recent publicity about DDT has got me scared. I'm expecting a baby in a few months and, until recently, planned on breast-feeding the child. But I've been reading that a mother's milk contains dangerously high levels of DDT.

One report even stated that if cow's milk had such high levels, it would be declared unsafe. Would I endanger my future child by nursing it?

ANSWER: A recent study has shown DDT content of mother's milk may exceed amounts of the pesticide permitted in cow's milk shipped in interstate commerce.

But weighing the benefits of breast-feeding against the unknown dangers of DDT contamination, I would still encourage you to nurse your child. And to join conservation groups working to control this kind of contamination.

Yogurt and Blindness

TOO MUCH DEPARTMENT: Most of us know that too much of almost anything can be unhealthy but this news will shake up many health food devotees. Yogurt can cause cataracts of the eyes! I know this news might get me banned from my favorite health food store but *Science* for June 12, 1970, reported that rats who ate only yogurt *all* developed cataracts.

Rats who were fed solely commercial yogurt seemed to enjoy the diet, grew normally and mated as zestfully as ever. But they all developed cataracts and young rats developed them earlier than adult rats. The Johns Hopkins investigators who conducted the study believe eye changes were caused by the high galactose content of commercially available yogurt.

Galactose is a type of sugar produced from a breakdown of milk carbohydrates. In high concentrations it is known to cause cataracts. But the galactose content of whole milk or of yogurt made from whole milk isn't that high ordinarily. So Curt Richter and James Duke, the authors of the study, checked into the way yogurt is prepared in our country. They found that butterfat is removed before milk is converted to commercial yogurt. Removing the butterfat produces a milk which has relatively more carbohydrates and hence more galactose. The milk produced, though, is too thin and watery so manufacturers add skim milk to improve the consistency, thus further increasing the percentage of galactose.

Richter and Duke say: "As evidence that cataracts produced by the yogurt diet result from its high content of galactose is the fact that cataracts produced by yogurt and galactose are clinically indistinguishable."

I've always wondered why people in health food stores seem to grope for their cups of yogurt. . . .

Dear Dr. Schoenfeld:

I learned through your column that processed yogurt may sometimes cause cataracts of the eyes. But my weakness is yogurt. Could you recommend the brand which would be least harmful?

ANSWER: Few humans would choose to eat an all-yogurt diet, and no case of cataracts in humans has ever been traced to excessive yogurt consumption.

The yogurt study was discussed only to emphasize that too much of anything may be harmful (almost anything, anyway). Immediately after writing that column I ate and thoroughly enjoyed a large serving of commercially prepared yogurt.

Gefilte Fish

Gefilte fish can be as lethal as it appears, according to an article in the October 13, 1969, *Journal of the A.M.A.* A Chicago housewife served a lunch of homemade gefilte fish to herself, a maid and her daughter-in-law. All were stricken with botulism, a particularly virulent type of food poisoning.

> The fish had been prepared from raw, unprocessed Great Lakes whitefish purchased in a supermarket. . . . Whole fish were ground at home to a fine paste . . . blended with raw eggs and onions, reground and made into patties approximately four inches in diameter. The patties were "simmered" for about four hours in a large open pot partially filled with water.

The gefilte fish was served cold with horseradish on toast (presumably, a piece of cooked carrot rested atop each piece). The housewife ate two pieces and died in a hospital five days later. Her maid, perhaps recognizing gefilte fish as somebody else's soul food, ate one piece, was hospitalized but survived. The daughter-in-law, who was seven months pregnant, ate only half a portion. She suffered dizziness, weakness, nausea, vomiting and a slight distortion of hearing but recovered without treatment. Two months later she gave birth to healthy twins.

Most gefilte fish in the United States is prepared from Great Lakes whitefish. Botulism organisms have been demonstrated in 9 percent of all fish caught in the Great Lakes. They are not killed off by horseradish, red or white.

As a medical student I learned about yet another danger of gefilte fish. Housewives sometimes ingest tapeworms while flavoring and tasting the uncooked fish meal.

Lest I be struck down by lightning, let me say that gefilte fish is not ordinarily poisonous. But the late Chicago matron who prepared the meal apparently didn't bring the fish to a boil.

Am I off the hook now, Mom, Aunt Ada, Aunt Ethel, Aunt Pearl, Aunt Sadie and Aunt Syd?

Conscientious Charter

Dear Dr. Schoenfeld:

I am writing to you in regard to my weight problem. I am 22, five feet six inches tall and I weigh 134 pounds. I would like to weigh 125 pounds. I have been as heavy as

145 pounds and really have had no trouble losing the first ten pounds but the second are a problem.

I perform fellatio on my boyfriend and my girlfriend told me the average caloric value of one ejaculation is 100.

Is it true that I am gaining calories by ingesting his semen? Should I keep an account of this and add it to my chart?

ANSWER: Dedicated medical researchers have found that the average ejaculation has a volume of 3 to 5 cubic centimeters—about a teaspoonful. Since the caloric value of a teaspoonful of pure sugar is only 18, it would seem likely that these felonies* committed with your boyfriend lead to a net caloric loss for both of you.

The Granola Papers

During the 1972 Republican National Convention my head research assistant and I were on a boat in the Bahamas ostensibly working on a book. Having spent more boyhood years in Miami Beach than I wished, I was curious about how tear gas would appear wafting down Collins Avenue. Late one afternoon, Susan Morehead and I walked down hotel row on our way to the Fontainebleau Hotel and a rendezvous with Dr. Raoul Duke, alias Hunter Thompson. Security was very tight so we disguised ourselves as freshly scrubbed Republican hippies. Susan said putting my long hair under a golfing cap was too obvious, but I did wear a short-sleeved sport shirt with vertical red, white, and blue stripes and a pair of white slacks saved from a summer as a ship's doctor.

* Fellatio is a crime punishable in California by prison terms of 1 to 14 years for each offense. Most other states have similar penalties.

We were also in disguise at the outset of our trip South. You see, I have a black Great Dane named Ahab and decided both of us would be happier if he came along. But Ahab had never been in an airplane before and I didn't care to have him flying for the first time freaked in a baggage compartment. The answer? A Seeing Eye dog is allowed to travel with its master. *Or mistress. So Susan Morehead put a white patch on her right eye and donned dark glasses while I constructed a huge harness for Ahab. My apprentice Sandy drove us to the airport, muttering something about "weird karma." We arrived at the San Francisco airport 15 minutes before our plane was due to leave—I think we were supposed to let the airline know in advance about flying with a guide dog. We didn't exactly fit the hijacker profile but harried National Airlines clerks and security personnel searched me and our luggage anyway. They didn't search Susan or Ahab.*

We were placed in first class seats next to an ominously whistling door marked "Barbara." My God, we were actually flying Barbara! Susan loved the trip, especially the times I had to cut up her food or lead her to the bathroom. The stewardesses were very solicitous. Our very high humor was marred only once, when the plane's captain left his cockpit to look us over.

"Which one of you is supposed to be blind?" asked the pilot, probably veteran of many scams, I thought.

"Why I am, sir," said Susan, looking not quite at him. She mentioned some unspeakable sailing accident and a chance for restored vision at the University of Miami's Bascomb Palmer Eye Institute.

"A Great Dane Seeing Eye dog?"

"Oh, he was ours before the accident and we trained him." (Ahab trained? He responds only to: Do you want to go [*anywhere*]*? or: Do you want to eat?)*

The captain seemed marginally convinced of Susan's condition, and said, "Well, I'm sure things will turn out all right."

After all, even if you doubt the story of two freaks traveling with a Great Dane Seeing Eye dog, what if the girl really is blind? The rest of our flight was uneventful except for Ahab snapping at a nervous stewardess and peeing on the cabin floor.

Uniformed guards in the Fontainebleau driveway were questioning three girls suspected of being demonstrators. Moments before, Jerry Rubin had been bounced from the hotel lobby. The guards looked at my tape recorder and waved us through as I started to reach for some nonexistent identification. Sitting on the hotel steps were several former Ant Farmers and Maureen Orth, then with Top Value TV (maybe you saw their choice coverage of the Democratic and Republican conventions—done with minuscule costs on Sony videotape equipment. Better than any network's). Their first words were not about the weirdness of the country's seat of power resting in Miami Beach, but the fall from grace of everyone's beloved cereal. Granola was just beginning to make itself known to New York City when a story in the August 20, 1972, *New York Times* reported the West Coast Granola Scandal. The *Times* had picked up the story from my column. We all consoled ourselves over the shattering revelations until the tall, lean figure of America's foremost political reporter lurched into sight. Slipping into the lobby we continued to the Poodle Room.

I could describe the demonstrators' encampment in Flamingo Park, young Republican convention cheerleaders and fans, or watching a beautiful, full Miami moon covered first with a wispy layer of clouds and then by billowing tear gas. But these events are insignificant compared with the granola story.

I don't know about you, but when I grew up most mornings included a brightly lettered package of a Kellogg's, General Mills', Nabisco's, or Post's dry cereal. My favorites then were cornflakes and Shredded Wheat—I was never convinced Wheaties would make me a champion. Sometimes nutritional contents would be listed, and I learned early that man does not live on dry cereal alone. Despite the stories, games, puzzles, and prizes I became indifferent toward breakfasts. Eggs didn't move me then.

While living in Berkeley, I first turned on to Swiss

Familia, a dry cereal which looked nutritious and tasted better than any of the BHA, BHT-preserved air-blown overrefined cereals I'd tasted till then. But sooner or later there comes the dreaded familia O.D. and it's never quite the same again. While visiting friends occupying a former firehouse, I sampled my first homemade granola, a delicious mixture that included plump pumpkin and sunflower seeds.

Granola packagers have multiplied in recent years due to growing consumer interest in health foods and recent Congressional hearings verifying most cereals were useful mainly as a vehicle for milk and fruit. In the San Francisco area, prepackaged granola appeared first in specialty health food stores, then Consumers Coop Markets, and finally in huge supermarket chains such as Safeway. There had clearly been an unsatisfied demand for prepared dry cereals that appeared healthful, pleased the taste and provided nutritional goodies not found in cruddy establishment brands.

Good old crunchy granola has now been a staple in my house for several years. I enjoy it with milk and fruit or sometimes over ice cream. Whether homemade or prepackaged, granola tastes better to me than any of the Kellogg's, General Mills' or Post's products. Of course I assumed granola was also far more nutritious than Wheaties or Cheerios. So did a lot of other people.

One morning I was reading the morning's mail and eating my favorite mixture of granola, sliced peaches and milk when my eye caught an article about granola in the *Consumers Coop News.* Helen Black, a Berkeley Coop home economist, noted sales of granola cereals, unaided by advertising, already amount to millions of dollars a year. Granolas, Ms. Black found, are usually mixtures of oats, nuts and seeds sweetened with brown sugar or honey and baked with oils. Sometimes other cereals, coconut, wheat germ or yeast are used. Ingredients must be listed by weight and the second heaviest ingredient is almost always the sweetener or oil. Helen Black calculated the nutritive value of her own favorite granola recipe. The ingredients were oats, brown sugar, sunflower seeds, oil, wheat germ, and salt. Equal weights of this mixture were compared with Cheerios,

Wheaties, Kix and the Coop's own Familia. She concluded granola had about the same amount of protein, iron, and thiamine as the other cereals. Granola excelled only in calories!

1-ounce portion	*calories*	*protein*	*iron*	*thiamin*
Granola	130	3.5gm*	1.3mgm**	195mcg***
Familia	110	2.7gm	1.2mgm	120mcg
Cheerios	112	3.8gm	1.2mgm	230mcg
Wheaties	104	2.8gm	1.7mgm	166mcg
Kix	112	2.5gm	1.2mgm	150mcg

*gm = gram **mgm = milligram ***mcg = microgram
28 grams = 1 ounce

A few weeks earlier a high school teacher had forwarded a question from his students about the healthfulness of granolas. His letter was answered in the next Hip Pocrates column with a summary of Ms. Black's findings. Response was swift and vehement. The usually friendly proprietor of our local health food store was rather surly during my next visit, even though a pound of her granola mix was among my purchases. A friend in Bolinas snarled to my secretary, "Dr. Hip may think he knows when he's been conned, but this time he's being double-conned."

Granola is homey, earthy and friendly. When we see it and taste it we *know* it's got to be good for us. Suggesting Cheerios are nutritionally equivalent to granola strikes most people I know as nothing less than blasphemy. Letters poured in. The most frequent comment concerned the density of granola vs. air-blown cereals. A bowl of granola does weigh several times more than the same size bowl of Cheerios, but the most reasonable way to compare food values is by weight, not volume.

Doktor:

Concerning your statistics on granola vs. All American breakfast: granola weighs in at 2–3 times as much as

Wheaties per unit volume. Nutritive value is greater in granola if raisins are included and it doesn't get soggy a few seconds after adding milk.

Dr. Joel Fort reminded me that "All-American" dry breakfast cereals originated with a Dr. Kellogg who had formulated a health food with famed curative powers. One of his patients, a man named Post, took the cure and liked it so well he devised his own health food cereal. The fluffed, preservative-ridden bastard descendants of their original formulas are hard to recognize today as health food. Grape-Nuts, at least, don't get soggy very quickly (if ever).

My correspondents seemed to forget I had but summarized Ms. Black's granola analysis:

Dear Dr. Schoenfeld:

I don't think you have told the whole story concerning the granola/Cheerios controversy. You only compare 3 categories and come to the conclusion that they are damn near identical. Even though I don't know the whole trip myself, I do know that your report is really incomplete. Perhaps a more detailed analysis is necessary, such as amino acids (what types and whether they are complete), Vitamin B complex (you probably know that niacin by itself don't do you much good) and how about all the other vitamins and minerals, carbohydrates and oils?

To end it all I think your article reflects a poor logic, no scientific technique, and a really big shaft put to all your readers. Perhaps you should publicly come clean, Doc, and straighten out your articles.

A call came from Alternative Features, a Berkeley group supplying news items to underground radio stations. The great granola controversy was about to spread further through the media. While they were taping our conversation my apprentice impishly sat on my lap. Since word was already going out to the underground that Dr. Hip was a suspected Un-Granolian, I gave way to an irresistible urge and told Alternative Features' tape recorder that male chauvinist Boss Schoenfeld was at the moment bouncing on his knee his "secretary," Sandy McLanahan, a fourth year medical student who helped in many ways—the least of which included her alleged typing skills.

On my last weekly radio program before leaving for a month in the Bahamas and Miami, most of the telephone calls concerned the great granola crunch. The most frequent reaction seemed to be anguish, followed by denunciations of Helen Black as an "Establishment Home Economist." As the program ended I turned to the producer and said I couldn't go on . . . there was nothing left to really believe in . . . good old crunchy granola exposed, etc. Sobbing, I left the airways. Some listeners called in later to find out if I *really* had been so emotionally distraught over the granola question.

After the ceremonial crowning of Nixon and Agnew, we returned to San Francisco immediately. Sandy was waiting with the (usually) trustworthy van. As we neared home I wanted only a bowl of granola, milk and fresh sliced peaches. Three weeks of forced abstinence! Sandy told me one of the granola companies had sent samples of their products. "And while you're testing the granola," she snickered, "you can go through the stack of granola letters." She had summarized the contents on their envelopes: "granola anger!," "granola has trace vitamins and minerals," "granola complaints" and "eggs beat out granola" were some.

Harmony Foods of Santa Cruz sent two packages of granola. One was called Mt. Kilamanjaro. "Remember," reminded the package, "these vitamins and minerals are naturally occurring—nature's own—not the synthetic additives found in most cereals."

One of the most difficult lessons learned in medical school was that body processes are not always logical. It seems logical that naturally occurring vitamins or "natural" vitamin pills are better utilized by the body than "synthetic" vitamins. But there is no evidence of any kind for this assumption. "Natural" and "organic" all too often are hollow slogans devoid of any real meaning.

Reading the package further I flashed back to the days of my shredded youth: "Very beautiful 22″ x 28″ full color detailed posters of the picture on this bag are available for $1.50 each." The posters *are* beautiful—at least I think so. One of them hangs on my kitchen wall today. Granola packagers don't yet offer decoder rings.

One reader introduced steak and eggs into the fast-thickening breakfast gruel:

Dear Dr. Schoenfeld:

Quality protein is by far the most costly part of human nutrition. Too many calories is the problem for most Americans. So, when the egg cholesterol delusion can be laid to rest, the best breakfast food nutritionally and economically becomes obvious from this table:

1 ounce	*calories*	*protein*	*iron*	*thiamin*	*approx. cost*
		gms	mg.	mcg.	
Granola	130	3.5	1.3	195	4¢
Cheerios	112	3.8	1.2	230	4.5¢
Wheaties	114	2.8	1.7	165	4¢
Kix	112	2.5	1.2	150	5¢
Steak	70	8.0	1.0	20	12¢
Eggs	45	3.5	.6	60	2¢

I agree that the relationship of cholesterol to heart disease is poorly established in humans.

Dear Dr. Schoenfeld,

There are granola and granola recipes! Combine dry ingredients: five cups of old fashioned oatmeal and one cup each of cut almonds, unrefined sesame seeds, sunflower seeds, shredded coconut, soy flour, powdered milk (preferably noninstant) and wheat germ.

Combine in separate bowl one cup honey and vegetable oil (not olive oil).

Combine dry and moist ingredients, spread on cookie sheets and bake 30 minutes or until lightly brown.

Pardon hurried letter. I am leaving for a vacation and making some granola to take along. Ha!

Let's examine another sacred belief here. There's certainly a vast difference between the taste of white sugar and the many available honeys. Almost always, I prefer honey as a sweetener. Is there a significant nutritional difference? If so, no one has yet produced any proof though many books and pamphlets claim refined sugar leaches out the body's vitamins and minerals, causes schizophrenia, and so on. A high carbohydrate diet does usually lead either to obesity or other forms of malnutrition. Obese people definitely have shortened life-spans and evidence is accumulating that high carbohydrate diets lead to diseases of the heart and blood vessels.

But look at honey compared with demon sugar:

1 ounce	*protein*	*calories*
Honey	0.1gm	98
Sugar	0	129

Surely, there is much yet to be learned about foods, but based on what we know now, there is little nutritional difference between honey and sugar. Honey does have trace amounts of B_1, B_2, niacin, C, calcium, magnesium, pantothenic acid, sodium, potassium, manganese, iron, copper, phosphorus, sulfur and chlorine. But the quantities are insignificant when compared with the body's needs.

Again and again we are told by the health food industry that sugar is bad and honey good. But too much honey will produce a severe case of lard-ass or granola-belly nearly as quickly as sugar.

We know woefully little about the ways we could use

food to treat disease or even maintain a state of optimum health. There's no doubt in my mind that people following certain diets feel healthier, higher and happier. But I don't know how much to attribute to faith and how much the diet. Fortunately for us humans, we can survive on a fantastic variety of foods. The man responsible for turning so many people on to vegetarianism, former LSD manufacturer Owsley Stanley, has eaten little but meat in the past 14 years. Unfortunately for us humans and other creatures, short-sighted economic measures cause our foods to be sprayed with toxins, injected with carcinogens, prepared only in forms acceptable to the greatest number of consumers, and preserved with poorly tested chemicals. Perhaps food is the key to the decreasing American life-span, perhaps not.

"Organic" food usually tastes better, probably contains fewer toxins, might be more nutritious, and almost always is more expensive. When it's available and feasible I choose it every time over processed food. At the same time, I know that people who buy all their food at Safeway or Food Fair and eat regularly at McDonald's or Howard Johnson's restaurants are just not dropping in the street like flies. I must acknowledge the possibility they will be as healthy as someone who shops only in health food stores. Do you disagree? On what basis?

But let's get back to the granola saga:

Dear Dr. Schoenfeld,

After reading about the hassle with "granola" vs. "cereal," I felt I ought to make a comment.

If Helen Black's findings are correct—that there are no nutritional differences between granola and other cereals, such as: Cheerios, Wheaties and Kix, then, no doubt, people are going to feel cheated. I mean if you can't trust good ole crunchy granola, then who can you trust?!

Maybe granola doesn't do much more for your body than other cereals, but it does great things for your psyche! I mean eating crunchy granola always seems to give me a "lift." Cheerios never gives me the "go-power" it claims to have in its advertisements. Granola "looks" healthier. It "feels" healthier. It's a very sensuous cereal! So I will continue, like others, to munch on my nutty granola, with nothing lost, but the trust in the last sane institution in this country! The granola makers!

Granolaism isn't a religious precept universally shared in the counterculture. Shelly Spindell, who runs Stinson Beach, California's Sunshine Gallery, gave this view:

"Granola? I don't eat granola. It gives me heartburn."

Nor do acknowledged health food experts agree that the granolas are good food sources. Martin Diamond, a former partner in Everybody's Foods, one of the largest health food stores in the San Francisco area, said,

Granola isn't a good food. It's like candy. I had my last bowl of granola a month ago late at night when I was seized by a sudden attack of hunger. I couldn't control myself. Granola's importance isn't nutritional but turning people on to foods without chemicals and preservatives.

Whether or not your favorite granola is Wheaties in natural food's clothing, we are certain to be deluged by many more brands before long. Waterbed manufacturers quickly figured the potential market. What's the market for breakfast cereals?

My letters on the subject contained a special delivery letter from John C. Watts, Ph.D., Vita-Crunch Foods' Director of Research & Development. His letter emphasized granola's density:

Looked at another way, to get the same amount of protein as contained in one serving of granola, it would be necessary to eat 2⅛ servings of Cheerios, 2⅝ servings of Wheaties and 3¾ servings of Kix.

A copy of the Vita-Crunch letter had been sent by them to home economist Helen Black. She replied directly to

Vita-Crunch, mailing me a carbon copy. She said comparing cereals on the basis of "commonly used portions" was not as accurate as a comparison based on weight. She added:

I wish companies such as yours would seriously consider reducing the sugars and fats in your formulas. People are more concerned now about nutrition than they have been for some years; perhaps now is the time to provide more nutritious products to meet their concern. Granola, without the sugar and oil, could be just such a product.

But without oil and a sweetener, granola tastes like cattle feed or worse. It's really awful. Almost anything can be sold if it's sweet enough. At the time Vita-Crunch sent me the special delivery letter, most of their products were actually made by Mrs. Alison's *Cookie* Company, Inc. (italics mine). Apparently, Mrs. Alison's Cookie Company knew a good (or at least sweet) thing when they saw one and decided to produce their own brand of granola. They sent a box containing 16 one-pound bags of "Mrs. Alison's Granola." The word *Cookie* was mysteriously absent from the packages. Listed as the first three ingredients were wheat, brown sugar, and oil.

After reading all the granola letters, many of which began something like "You call that granola? Granola should contain the following ingredients . . . , " the time seemed opportune to spoon into yet another area of the boundless opportunities for Granola Research. Members of my research staff made the following report:

Usually we eat granola in the morning. What if we altered our minds a bit—by having granola in the evening! So prepared, we bent to our task, savoring each morsel of coconut, sunflower seeds, oats and raisins. The taste, we found, is important, yes, but not more so than its texture. An entire school of psychology is based on ways people chew their food. Granola gives a very satisfying crunch pleasing to the jaws and teeth.

Crunch! You pasty pale overrefined imperialist dry cereal lackeys! Crunch! Cheerios were never so chewy. Crunch! Rice Crispies crackle and pop but meld with the milk. Crunch! Grape-Nuts are petrified. Crunch! We don't need BHT in Raisin Bran. Crunch! They were champions in spite of Wheaties. Crunch! We get our Kix other ways now. Crunch! Crunch! Crunch!

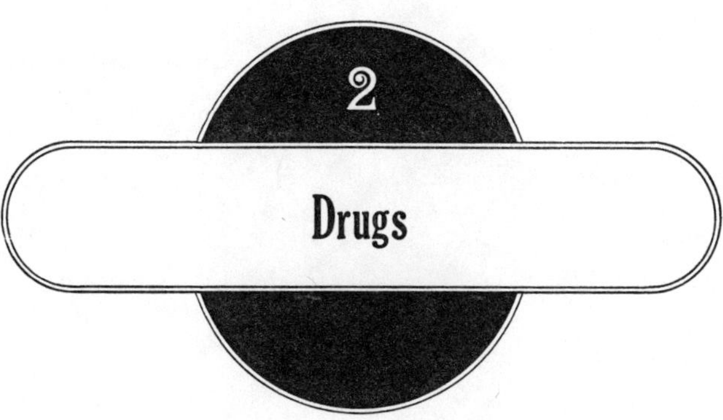

2

Drugs

The "Drug Problem"

In 1971 President Richard M. Nixon spoke before the annual meeting of the American Medical Association, which now represents a minority of physicians in the United States. Nixon stated that drug abuse was "public enemy number one," thereby giving that problem precedence over the rising crime rate, the shaky state of the nation's economy and, most importantly, the illegal and immoral war in Indochina.

Certainly drug abuse is a disturbing and important public health problem, but closer to "public enemy number one" is a mentality that purports to help people by passing increasingly stringent, counterproductive drug laws. More dangerous than any known result of drug abuse is the increasing control over medicine wielded by the Justice Department:

> The [Justice] Department personnel need only decide that some compound doesn't conform to their view of what constitutes a safe drug, and that's the end of that. The right of decision has been taken out of the hands of the medical scientist.
>
> Francis Braceland, M.D.,
> Editor of the *American Journal of Psychiatry*
> (*Hospital Tribune,* February 23, 1970)

Other "cures" far worse than the disease they purport to cure are "no-knock laws," unannounced searches of school lockers and the use of informers in public schools and colleges.

The use of marijuana by millions of Americans has finally prompted their government to authorize some research with this drug. But virtually banned are legal experiments with other mind-affecting substances that might help man understand better his mental processes. Recently I heard a physician say "drugs are only for sick people." Is this a fact? Or does it reflect a common but narrow viewpoint?

What are the best ways of preventing harm through the use and abuse of drugs? The first and most important step would be abolishing criminal penalties for their possession and use. The youth culture is hardly united on most domestic issues but regarding this area of personal freedom they speak with one voice—FREE ALL DRUG PRISONERS. The punitive approach to drug abuse has never proven effective. An alcoholic jailed hundreds of times heads directly for a bottle on being released from jail.

A second step would be establishment of street drug analysis centers wherever illicit drug use is found. When samples of street drugs are analyzed they usually differ from claims made for them by drug dealers. "LSD" is found to have additives like PCP, "mescaline" proves to be STP or LSD, hashish is shown to contain generous amounts of camel dung, etc. Publication of street drug analyses has been recommended since 1970 by the Canadian Commission on the Nonmedical Use of Drugs. Acting on its recommendation, the Drug Information Foundation in Amsterdam, the Do It Now Foundation in Los Angeles and other groups have established street drug testing centers.

Drug information, like other areas touching on moral and sociological issues, must necessarily reflect the philosophies of informants. For example, the July 26, 1971, issue of the *Journal of the A.M.A.* featured an article titled "Testicular Choriocarcinoma in LSD Users." The report concerns two young men with cancer of the testicles who had used LSD at some point prior to developing the malignancy. Since millions of young men have used LSD, it is not surprising that some of them might develop cancer, just as some young men never using LSD also develop testicular cancer. If the article pointed to a noncontroversial substance it would undoubtedly have been returned promptly to the authors as a wild theory unsupported by any valid evidence. But the article was printed. What are the implications of the American Medical Association's publishing an article based on such flimsy information?

We might learn something from the old show business sayings, "any publicity is good publicity," "every knock a boost," as we consider the endless flow of drug abuse film and TV documentaries, newspaper articles, dope forums, etc. Apart from the fact that most such information is misleading, recent studies demonstrated ill-conceived drug education programs can actually *increase* drug use—and presumably, drug abuse.

Germaine Greer made a shrewd observation on efforts to curb drug misuse in the United States. While riding a subway in New York City she noticed a large attractive color poster with gleaming reproductions of tablets, capsules, syringes and needles. At the bottom of the placard was the word, "DON'T!" But the message clearly imparted was "DO!"

Drugs possess no moral qualities. They are not intrinsically good, bad, holy or evil. They do produce effects and side effects. Knowing these effects and teaching them in a credible manner (drug education, in other words) is our best hope for preventing drug abuse.

Long before the widespread illegal use of drugs we were unmistakably a drug culture. Consider the daily intake of drugs by a typical family as observed by a child. He sees his parents groping for coffee and cigarettes as soon as they awaken. Use of these drugs continues through the day. The effects of tobacco are now well known and if anyone doubts coffee is used as a drug just compare sales of decaffeinated and caffeine-containing brands.

Our hypothetical child watches his mother use tranquilizers and perhaps amphetamines if she is overweight or tired. When father returns from work he immediately downs a couple of martinis. Perhaps he's had one or two drinks with lunch as well. Sleep may be induced with the aid of barbiturates. By the time children enter school they are aware that drug use is both encouraged and freely practiced by their elders. They know drug use is considered morally right by most Americans.

Drug education in this context must aim at presenting known scientific facts. If information about drugs is lacking, this must also be admitted.

An interesting study might be conducted in college dispensaries comparing visits for acute alcohol intoxication with visits for untoward marijuana reactions during the past ten years. Studies of this sort will be needed if we are ever to have reliable data on the nature and scope of the "drug problem."

Recently I received the following letter:

For the nine months of my pregnancy I refrained from taking any drugs, psychedelic or other. Now that my baby has arrived, I would like to resume taking acid and mescaline. But I plan to breast-feed for at least 6 months.

Will these drugs reach my baby through my milk and, if so, will they come through strongly enough to affect him? I could express the milk before taking the drugs but how long would they remain in my milk supply? Please advise.

This is one of the most commonly asked questions received in my mail. The mother is willing to risk her own health but not her baby's and this concern, it seems to me, is not being shared by those who could authorize and conduct a study of this and related questions in laboratory animals. Restrictions on legitimate psychedelic drug research do harm not only because such information might be beneficial to psychiatrists and others, but because lack of information may cause users of these drugs unwittingly to harm themselves or their children. The advice I give is that no one yet knows whether LSD, mescaline or marijuana enter breast milk but pending more information it's best not to take a chance.

My experience has been that people cannot be dissuaded from drug use by moral preachments, threats or imprisonment. Drug education seems to me the single most important method in preventing drug abuse but is usually viewed narrowly and conducted poorly.

Stanley F. Yolles, M.D., director of the National Institute of Mental Health believes mandatory jail sentences should be eliminated in connection with the use and sale of all drugs, including heroin. Testifying before the House Crime Committee, Dr. Yolles said, "I am convinced that the social and psychological damage caused by incarceration is in many cases far greater to the individual and to society than was the offense itself . . . It is time to change from a prosecution to a public health approach in dealing with drug abuse and especially in cooling the marijuana problem . . ."

Resolution of the "drug problem" will be consciously or unconsciously resisted by many divergent groups. Criminal organizations which profit through drug trafficking hardly welcome legal use of drugs which now bring substantial incomes. Individual drug dealers, who constitute one of the nation's fastest growing "professions," often enjoy, even more than the money gained, the adventure of such a blatant antiestablishment activity. What about the many government employees of agencies involved with drug abuse problems? Has there ever been a bureaucrat who welcomed a reduction of his power and budget? The "drug police" (a term coined by Joel Fort, M.D.) are not the only state-supported agents who will lose should drug abuse cease being a matter of public concern. What about the thousands employed by the billion dollar drug education and rehabilitation industries? After all, when directors of methadone maintenance clinics tell us their patients must be kept addicts forever they imply their clinic staffs will be also forever maintained and that federal grants will continue always.

Even more important than drug education, regulation and rehabilitation in combating drug abuse is the correction of individual and societal problems leading people to stupefy or destroy themselves with drugs rather than face what we usually call reality. I refer to intolerably dull educational programs, racial tensions, economic instability and senseless warfare wrought against the will of the people.

Writing in *The Journal of Social Issues* (Vol. 27, No. 3, 1971), psychologist William H. McGlothlin notes:

> One of the consistent historical observations about drug using behavior is that excessive use flourishes during periods of social upheaval. Where family, community, and cultural structure are strong, abuse is low; when wars, massive migrations from rural to urban settings, unemployment, and breakdown of family influence occur, abuse tends to be high. In short, lack of structure, discipline, and involvement are conducive to patterns of excessive drug use. If one projects a future society in which large segments of the population are unemployed or otherwise alienated and uninvolved, then a high rate of drug abuse can be anticipated.

Marijuana

My first experience with marijuana occurred when I was fourteen years old. A relative active in show business was visiting my family and one night I borrowed his jacket for a "heavy date." I found a hand-rolled, funny-looking cigarette in the right-hand coat pocket.

School hygiene classes had shown movies warning of the dangers of "reefers," something I vaguely associated with old newspaper photos of actor Robert Mitchum doing time in a Los Angeles jail. Only two people in my high school were even suspected of using marijuana at the time. When

I asked my relative if the strange cigarette I'd found was marijuana, he simply told me yes. Previously, I had tried to inhale tobacco with disastrous results (gagging, choking), and perhaps this caused me to have no interest in smoking the first "reefer" I had seen.

Later, in Berkeley, I had some folk-singer friends who were the first people I'd ever seen actually using marijuana. One of the interesting things I noticed was that soon after they smoked a few jays someone would be sent out for ice cream and chocolate syrup, rushing past the window of Toni Brown (*Joy of Cooking*) who lived in the same funky building.

I always refused their offer to turn on (partially because I'd just received my medical license), but I usually felt euphoric when I left my friends' low-ceilinged apartment. I'd either inhaled the room smoke or gotten contact highs—I'll never know. By that time I did know most of what passed for information about marijuana was false. The weed hadn't made my friends weird. They had always been weird.

During the spring and summer of 1963, I wandered through Europe, after completing my internship and serving as a staff physician in a county outpatient clinic and geriatric hospital in order to save some money for my travels. Outside the Athens American Express office I met a girl I'd known in Berkeley. She was on her way to a small island named Skyros, where poet Rupert Brooke once lived. We decided to meet there in a week. To the delight of several other American friends on the island, Mickey arrived bearing a large chunk of hashish. She mixed some of it with tobacco, rolled a cigarette and passed it around. I coughed and hacked as I always do when inhaling tobacco. Whether it was the tobacco or hash that got me stoned, I soon found myself very interested in wind-blown leaves scudding slowly across the patio in brilliantly clear Greek sunlight.

When I returned to the United States that fall I enrolled in Yale's Master of Public Health program. Whenever possible I'd leave New Haven. If I drove or took the train to New York City, I'd often visit a girl (from Berkeley again) who many times had urged me to try marijuana. Every reputable source I had read to that time, including pharmacology texts and my own observations and limited experience, had convinced me the greatest harm marijuana could cause was legal, not medical. But basically, I was driven to pot by New Haven.

Jennifer drew the blinds to her second-floor, West 79th Street apartment and proceeded to teach me how to inhale. Well, the experiment was a success. I learned to inhale and got righteously stoned in the process. I think I experienced almost all the varied effects of marijuana that evening, including ravenous hunger, euphoria and paranoia (I was afraid someone might peer beneath the window shade—of course in New York it might easily have happened). Jennifer had a scroll with an Oriental temple rubbing mounted on the kitchen wall, and for some reason I decided it was necessary to glue a Jan Heebler almond cookie beneath it. But there was no glue. So I made some paste from flour and water, something I hadn't done since grade school. The gooey mixture felt good on my fingers, too. For all I know that almond cookie remains on the wall.

Legal experimentation with marijuana is presently conducted in several American university medical schools. As a subject of research studies in the Langley Porter Neuropsychiatric Institute of San Francisco's University of California Medical Center, I learned firsthand the official methods used to add to our growing body of knowledge of cannabis. I also learned strong dope is available through local narcotics bureaus. My experience with marijuana has included treating patients who had unpleasant experiences with the drug. As a staff physician with the student health service of the University of California at Berkeley, I saw several students with panic reactions, usually after their first usage of marijuana.

The letters and answers which follow cover the broad range of reactions to cannabis. Untoward reactions are greatly overrepresented in order to demonstrate more clearly that no drug is completely safe for everyone. Many long-time heads now use the drug less frequently or not at all. Often friends have said:

"Marijuana doesn't get me high anymore."

"Marijuana brings me down."

"It makes me tired when it wears off."

"I can't do my work when I'm stoned."

Perhaps the reasons are psychic, perhaps metabolic. Perhaps the quality of the grass is involved. On the other hand, there will probably be many who'll continue to use the drug all their lives without noticeable detriment.

One thing seems certain. Attempts to regulate private behavior and thought through tyrannical laws will ultimately fail.

International Concerns

Dear Dr. Hip:

I am a Nigerian, 21 and three-fourths years old with West African School Certificate Grade 2.

Earlier this year, my mother and father caught me smoking pot. My mother started weeping. She said marijuana smoking causes permanent damage to the brain.

She referred to the many Nigerian street lunatics with the allusion that it is the dope that makes them become insane.

I started smoking it in the secondary school and that is some 5 years ago. I haven't experienced any brain fatigue but now I am seriously afraid.

1) *Can marijuana cause brain damage?*
2) *Can pot smoking cause lung cancer, heart disease or any other deadly disease?*
3) *Is it true that smoking marijuana can render me childless?*

ANSWER: The street "lunatics" in Lagos may be the equivalent of our alcoholic skid row bums. Marijuana seems to be less dangerous than alcohol for most people but, like any drug, can be abused. Marijuana grown in your country is very strong due to favorable weather conditions.

Because extensive marijuana research has not been encouraged in my country despite its use by millions of Americans, physicians don't know enough about the drug's potential benefits and possible dangers. However, I'll try to answer your questions:

1) Marijuana is not known to cause brain damage. But a study published in the May 3, 1969, issue of *Nature* confirmed the observations of most users that speech and short-term memory are temporarily affected by the drug. Doctors Andrew Weil and Norman Zinberg, who reported one of the first American scientific studies of marijuana in humans in 1968, also conducted the *Nature* study.

   Weil and Zinberg found that instant or immediate memory was affected by marijuana. The "principle manifestations of this speech difficulty are simply the forgetting of what one is going to say next and a strong tendency to go off on irrelevant tangents because the line of thought is lost." Most marijuana users, incidentally, seem to enjoy this effect.

2) Pot smoking is not known to cause lung cancer or any other disease. But widespread marijuana use has occurred in this country only for a few years. Lung cancer caused by cigarettes takes many years to develop.

   There is every reason to believe that chronic inhalation of marijuana smoke may be harmful to the lungs. We cannot accumulate the necessary statistics while criminal penalties face marijuana users.

3) Marijuana is not known to render people childless. On the contrary, the drug enhances sexual excitement if the individuals are so inclined.

   The universal use of drugs such as alcohol and marijuana indicates to me that man enjoys, perhaps needs, to change his mind at times. But as a physician I want to be aware of all possible consequences arising from drug usage.

Shortly after the preceding letter and answer appeared, I received a note from Dr. Joshua Lederberg, Stanford University's Nobel Prize-winning geneticist. He questioned the statement that marijuana "enhances sexual excitement if the individuals are so inclined."

Memo from: J. Lederberg
Genetics Department
Stanford University
Stanford, California

To: Dr. Schoenfeld—

Unless this is really a hard fact (which I strongly doubt), this strikes me as a rather irresponsible incitement.

At most, is not the most plausible statement that cannabis may relieve unconscious inhibitions (not unlike alcohol)?

My answer to Dr. Lederberg was that I do not think marijuana causes sexual excitement. But patients, acquaintances and friends have invariably reported marijuana increases sexual enjoyment if they are already turned on. If a couple is turned off to each other, marijuana seems to increase the turnoff.

I also told Dr. Lederberg I did not believe marijuana and alcohol affect sex in the same way. Alcohol has long been employed in seduction ("alcohol dissolves the superego") but few people would claim this drug increases physical sensitivity. Large amounts of alcohol, in fact, commonly cause impotence.

A scientific study of this question will be difficult to structure. Perhaps readers could suggest ways of presenting the hard facts desired by Dr. Lederberg. A hirsute Englishman recommended a Stanford coed and a joint.

Grass and Impotence

Dear Dr. Schoenfeld:

The 1971–72 A.M.A. president, Dr. Wesley W. Hall, stated he knew of a study which showed pot smoking causes impotence and birth defects. He said it would make a man of 35 sexually like a man of 70.

I doubt the validity of this report from my personal experiences. In fact I find balling better when I'm stoned. Anyway, I'd like your opinion.

ANSWER: No drug should be taken during pregnancy unless advised by a physician but if marijuana caused a significant number of birth defects the thalidomide disaster of a few years ago would seem small by comparison. Dr. Hall later said he'd been "misquoted." He also said that even if his statement wasn't true, perhaps it stopped some people from using marijuana. A curious statement from the leader of this nation's largest physicians' organization.

When I spoke with my brother the psychiatrist about this alleged link between marijuana, birth defects and impotency, he said, "They really know how to hit where it hurts." The A.M.A. seems determined to play out its role as dinosaur.

Germ Killer Weed?

Dr. Schoenfeld,

Through the entire spectrum of literature on marijuana, nothing has had more color than the theory: Grass has antiseptic properties; it kills germs. Could you please comment.

ANSWER: Marijuana does have weak antibiotic properties against some types of bacteria. If you're lost in the woods with an infected wound and a stash of grass, don't smoke it. Make a moist poultice instead and apply it to the wound.

Can't Get High

Dear Dr. Schoenfeld:

This may sound ridiculous, but I swear it's the truth: on four different occasions I have been to parties where a goodly amount of grass was smoked and everyone else gets turned on but me. It's obviously not the quality of the grass since everyone else got high—and it couldn't be a put-on because they were different groups of people.

Have you heard of this happening before? What can I do about it? I've been instructed by experts, so that's not the problem either. My only clue—I take 10 mgms of Librium 3 times per day under doctor's orders (for neurodermatitis). Could that turn me off?

ANSWER: There are two possible answers to your "problem." One is the great variation of responses to drugs. The spectrum of human experience is such that some people will have no reaction when almost everyone else having the same quantity will be under (or over) the table. Your friends have no doubt told you, in addition, that the effects of marijuana must be anticipated and learned.

But the most likely cause for your not feeling the effects of marijuana is the daily use of a tranquilizer. Bad psychological reactions to marijuana are rare, but when they do occur they are often treated with Librium or other tranquilizers in order to bring the patient down.

A Rough Blend

Dear Dr. Schoenfeld:

In sharing an occasional joint with some young people during the last few weeks, I have been horrified to discover that grass is sometimes massively adulterated with tobacco. This is apparently a recent development but the kids seem unaware or uncaring about it.

Middle-Aged Worrier

ANSWER: Many ask whether addictive drugs such as heroin are commonly added to marijuana in order to hook the user. People are usually introduced to heroin through their "friends" rather than through plots of the Mafia or other arms of organized crime. Besides, lacing marijuana with more expensive drugs is usually economically unfeasible.

I suppose some small-time, pea-brained dealers might add tobacco to marijuana—fraud and greed are not confined to the Establishment.

Hide the Stash

Dr. Frederic Frye, a Berkeley veterinarian, recently published an article in the *Journal of the American Veterinary*

Medical Association reporting the case of a puppy accidentally poisoned by marijuana.

The nine-week-old female spaniel was brought to his clinic in a semiconscious state by its three masters who did not know the cause of its illness. Within the dog's mouth, plant material was found lodged between the teeth, gums and cheeks. The material consisted of seeds, leaves and stem fragments.

On discovering the plant substances, the pup's three owners responded strangely: one grinned, one giggled, and the third wept. The dog was treated with stimulants and an emetic which caused it to vomit approximately one ounce of cannabis sativa. Ten hours after treatment the dog seemed completely straight.

Local veterinarians report that many pets are fed marijuana cookies or brownies by their masters. (Some animals have also been given LSD or shot up with heroin or methedrine.) Usually, the weight of the dog is not taken into account. Though animals vary in their reactions to drugs depending on species—it makes no sense to give a 15-pound dog the same quantity of a drug used by a 150-pound man—even if it made sense to give animals these drugs, and it doesn't.

Puppies and small children seem to have a knack for finding and eating large quantities of potentially dangerous substances (such as aspirin). Cache all drugs, insecticides, kerosene, etc., in places where curious small creatures cannot possibly get to them.

Drug Reaction

Dear Dr. Schoenfeld:

The other night I smoked some grass, not any more than usual. But this time I passed out for a few minutes and don't remember a thing. Worse than that my legs and rear end sweated immensely. I was so sopping wet that it was necessary to change both pants and underwear. I did not have anything alcoholic to drink.

Could you please give me some kind of reason for this

happening? Will it happen again? Should I see a doctor? I am worried about it as it was an awful experience.

ANSWER: Perhaps you smoked tobacco rather than marijuana. The symptoms you described can occur when someone inhales tobacco deeply, especially the first time. But some people have a similar reaction to smoking marijuana. It is also possible, though unusual, to develop an allergy to marijuana which could cause these symptoms.

Certainly you should be checked by a physician—tell him about this experience and your past drug usage. He could give you some helpful medical advice.

Another Fainting Spell

Dear Dr. Schoenfeld:

To be blunt, I'm scared. I was smoking some grass about 3 weeks ago and I started to feel dizzy. Next thing I remember is waking up on the floor and being told I'd been unconscious about 7 minutes.

This wouldn't bug me so much except that I can remember coming close to blacking out 4 times when I was younger: in preschool, at the blackboard in a writing class in the third grade, at confirmation when I was about 11, and at a wedding when I was about 15.

All of the times I've fainted were when I was very uptight, like wanting to be somewhere else, so I've usually figured it's just some psychological trip—like I shut myself off when I'm threatened.

Do you think seeing a head doctor would do any good? I can't afford a private doctor.

ANSWER: Recently I treated a student for bizarre symptoms after he'd smoked marijuana from a waterpipe with a group of friends. He had been noncommunicative for several hours before being brought to the hospital.

When I first saw him he was lying on the floor face down trying to crawl away from his friends. Then he crawled into a corner under a stretcher, obviously terrified. He couldn't be talked down (as most people can on bad trips), so I had the nurse give him a tranquilizer by injection. Within a few minutes, *long before the effects of the tranquilizer could have taken effect,* he was responding in a normal manner.

The student told me similar experiences had occurred before he had ever used marijuana. I referred him to a neurologist to determine whether any physical cause could be found for this behavior.

You should have a thorough physical examination soon. Perhaps you are eligible for private medical care through one of the welfare programs even if you are otherwise self-supporting. Call your county welfare department to learn whether you qualify as a "medical indigent."

Spicing or Spiking

Dear Dr. Schoenfeld:

Last weekend, a gourmet chef visited our house and prepared a delicious cold rice salad. Amongst the spices in the salad dressing was a generous dash of marijuana.

He told no one about this recipe until the dozen of us were on our third helpings. By that time, it was obvious that our nonsmoking household had been affected very pleasantly.

When I told other people about the meal, many of them said that pot can only affect one through smoking. Who is right?

ANSWER: You are. But the gourmet chef was wrong.

Marijuana is certainly effective when taken by mouth and more active when heated. That's why cookie and brownie (Alice B. Toklas's variety) baking has become so popular recently. Effects of ingested marijuana don't become apparent for an hour or so and then last four or five hours.

Secretly adding any drug to food or drink is dangerous. Even though marijuana is relatively nontoxic, an innocent brownie muncher might become frightened and panicky if he didn't know the cause of his trip.

Some physicians believe smoking marijuana is preferable

to eating it because inhaled marijuana is effective within minutes, allowing the smoker to control his high. If the drug is ingested, more of it may be taken than desired. On the other hand, marijuana smoke often feels irritating to the lungs, though much more pot is usually necessary for this effect than tobacco.

Grass and Mental Illness

Dear Dr. Schoenfeld:

What's the advisability of turning on someone who had a nervous breakdown years ago and had a bout with paranoia?

She seems to be on her feet now. Would she flip out on grass?

ANSWER: She might. Psychotic reactions following the use of marijuana are rare but they do occur. Paranoid feelings under the influence of marijuana are common, depending usually on the prestoned state of the individual. If your friend were with strangers in unfamiliar surroundings, the chances for an unpleasant experience would be greatly increased.

Peer Pressure

Dear Dr. Hip Pocrates:

I am very concerned about the effects marijuana smoking has upon me. Almost always I have a bad time: I get very frightened and paranoid.

Often I can't talk and at times I start to shake. I feel very unconfident. This has caused me to shy away from hip people which is not where it's really at these days.

When turned on with grass I get a very fast, pulsating (about strobe light speed) vibration. With acid or speed I do not notice the vibration or fear and helplessness. Any information you can give will be greatly appreciated.

ANSWER: Marijuana often produces feelings of paranoia but the symptoms you describe should cause you to stop using the drug now. People who are truly hip won't put you down because you don't use marijuana.

Allergic Reaction?

Dear Dr. Hip:

Please tell me if it is possible that certain people can have a kind of allergic reaction to smoking grass. It seems that too often when I smoke I get a kind of suffocating feeling. As silly as it sounds, I feel that I have to "burp" and I can't, then pressure seems to build up. If medically this is impossible then I guess I have to come to terms with this on a psychological basis.

ANSWER: Allergy to marijuana is possible or you may be swallowing rather than inhaling the smoke.

Eye Irritation

Dear Dr. Hip Pocrates:

I have been smoking marijuana with a friend of mine (not steadily) for four years. We both suffer from eye irritation every time we smoke it. This irritation seems serious enough (extremely red, swollen and sensitive to light) to raise the question of whether or not it is possible to be allergic to marijuana smoke, or if it is a side effect occurring to a few unfortunate users.

Only a few of the many people we know that smoke marijuana seem to reach the point of eye irritation that we do. Since I have gotten contact lenses, about two years ago, it has become increasingly unbearable. My friend does not wear contact lenses yet her eyes become just as badly irritated.

When we use eye drops, it gives very temporary relief of perhaps 30 seconds, and it must be reapplied every five minutes. It's not very convenient, to put it mildly.

Rather than give up the pleasure of smoking dope, is there any prevention, cure or possibility of this being an allergy?

ANSWER: Marijuana commonly causes red eyes due to a widening of blood vessels in the white of the eye. The severe symptoms you describe are unusual but could be caused by this effect. Allergy to marijuana is another possibility but you'd probably have other symptoms such as wheezing or sneezing.

See your family physician, an ophthalmologist, or go to the nearest free clinic. But do not use contact lenses over irritated eyes.

Marijuana and Studying

Dear Dr. Schoenfeld:

If you were a freshman student in college and you really didn't dig, let's say algebra, would you smoke grass moderately, heavily or not at all (I hope not!) to help you study better?

ANSWER: I doubt very much whether marijuana would help your studies of algebra. If you don't dig doing something, chances are you'll like it even less under the influence of grass.

Besides, marijuana impairs short-term memory.

One well-known illustration of short-term memory impairment is the phenomenon of someone under the influence of marijuana beginning a long sentence and, by the time he reaches the end, forgetting what he started out to say (What was that?—secy's note). A student going to class stoned on grass might be less likely to remember the lecture than one going there straight. No evidence has yet indicated that marijuana affects long-term memory.

High Tar Count

Dear Dr. Schoenfeld:

Marijuana is often weighted down with sugar, as I'm sure many smokers know. The obvious purpose seems to be to give as little grass as possible for the weight of the kilo or lid.

I understand that sugar, when smoked, turns to tar in

the lungs which can easily and rapidly cause emphysema. What is your opinion of this? Personally, I am going back to baking brownies.

ANSWER: Several readers have asked about sugar found in their marijuana. But my informants tell me its purpose is neither to add weight nor to sweeten the effect. Sugar or sugar-containing soft drinks are sometimes used to make the leafy particles stick together when marijuana is compressed into kilogram bricks and illegally imported into the country.

Try burning a cube or lump of sugar. The black chunk of carbon which results will give you an idea of the effect on your lungs of smoking sugar. Even when marijuana hasn't been sugared, its smoke leaves a tarry residue. No one knows at this time whether marijuana smoke is more or less harmful to the lungs than an equivalent amount of tobacco smoke.

Moth-Brained Dealer

Dear Dr. Schoenfeld:

Our last kilo contained hundreds of chips of crushed mothballs. We have heard tell of grass cured in mothballs, but had never seen any before. The grass had a peculiar medicinal odor and a metallic taste.

Could there be any possible harm in smoking or swallowing chips too small to see?

ANSWER: Your friendly dealer may lose a lot of customers. Mothballs usually contain 100 percent naphthalene. Naphthalene is fatal in quantities of 2 grams for children and 5 to 15 grams for adults when ingested at one sitting. The drug is also quite toxic when inhaled.

Some of the symptoms of naphthalene intoxication are headache, confusion, excitement, nausea, and sometimes sweating and vomiting. Death occurs when red blood cells distintegrate causing kidney damage from cellular material released by the lysed red cells.

Those suspecting they have ingested or inhaled naphthalene should see a physician in order to have a complete blood count.

Brain Damage in Washington

Dear Dr. Schoenfeld:

A recent newspaper article reported Pentagon researchers had found marijuana in large doses caused irreversible brain damage in laboratory animals. Is this just propaganda?

ANSWER: Any substance in sufficient quantity, including water, can cause irreversible damage to the body. Previous extensive studies of marijuana, including the British Hemp Commission and LaGuardia Reports, found no impairment with moderate usage. Many of us, though, have suspected for a long time a brain damage epidemic in the Pentagon.

Reverse Tolerance

Dear Dr. Schoenfeld:

I'm a graduate student in sociology. Within the last year I have become almost a daily user of marijuana, averaging about four to six joints per week and oftentimes more. I vaguely recall reading an article a couple of months ago in which a research team collected evidence to indicate "a reverse tolerance." Among chronic marijuana users it took less to get high than for occasional users, apparently because of residues that remained in the system.

With myself and a few close friends it seems that the above described phenomenon at times applies but then there are other instances where it seems to be the opposite. For example, tonight after abstaining for a week it took less to get ripped than it normally does. In your opinion which process do you think is at work?

ANSWER: Components of marijuana apparently do remain in the body for several days after use but whether or not they have anything to do with "reverse tolerance" is unknown. Most experienced marijuana users have noticed that sometimes they require less weed to get high while at other times they can munch many brownies or smoke up a storm without feeling very much besides fatigue. I think several factors must be considered including the quality of marijuana, the length of time a particular batch is used, and where your head is at.

The "contact high" is well known, that is a person entering a room of people stoned on grass may get high just by being with them. Reverse tolerance may be a psychological as well as a pharmacological phenomenon.

Grass and Glaucoma

Dear Dr. Schoenfeld:

Is grass or acid contraindicated for people with glaucoma? My mother-in-law has glaucoma, controlled by pupil contracting drops, and I'm wondering if it's safe to turn her on.

ANSWER: There is now definite evidence that cannabis lowers pressure within the eyeball. Marijuana or one of its components might well be useful for treating glaucoma.

Swollen Heads

Dear Dr. Schoenfeld:

Can using hashish affect the ears in such a way that sometimes it feels like the ears are stuffed with wax when they are actually clean?

ANSWER: Cannabis products, such as hashish and marijuana, can cause enlargement of small blood vessels and swelling of mucous membranes. Users commonly notice reddening of the eyes and stuffy noses. The same effect could also cause swelling and narrowing of the Eustachian tubes (which run between the mouth and ears), thus causing a feeling of the ears being stuffed.

A Diabetic Head

Dear Dr. Hip Pocrates:

I think you are being entirely unfair in advising diabetics not to use marijuana.

I am a 28-year-old juvenile diabetic using insulin for almost 10 years—am also an R.N. I have been smoking grass for about a year and have found that it neither increases nor decreases the blood sugar.

But I believe you should tell all diabetics whether they are drinking alcohol, smoking grass or taking a psychedelic drug to make sure they have enough to eat and continue to eat during their high. I can't think of anything worse than a stoned diabetic in an insulin reaction—it would be impossible to recognize the symptoms.

I would encourage a diabetic to take precautions against an insulin reaction even to the point of overeating. I'd rather spill sugar in my urine than have an insulin reaction. The diabetic should also make sure the brothers and sisters whom they smoke with can recognize an insulin reaction.

Distorted Reality

Dear Dr. Schoenfeld:

I'm writing about "Effects of Marijuana on Adolescents and Young Adults," which was published in the April 19, 1971 issue of the A.M.A. Journal. *After reading it over a few times, I found that it was hardly worth the paper it was printed on.*

The authors singled out 38 marijuana smoking psychiatric patients and attempted to prove that their problems were the result of using marijuana. If the research was to be truly scientific, the authors would have gotten rid of all but one variable—the use of marijuana. This report appeared to be like the faulty information of the '30s which prompted the enactment of the severely harsh marijuana laws.

Am I right?
S.P.
Humboldt State College

ANSWER: Articles about drugs in the *Journal of the A.M.A.* often seem to reflect official A.M.A. policies rather than scientific knowledge. One pharmacologist who agreed with your interpretation of "Effects of Marijuana on Adolescents and Young Adults" thought the authors should be jailed!

Psychiatrists tend to forget that drug users they treat are not representative of the general drug-using population. Even though this study violated scientific principles, the *A.M.A. News* ran a banner headline on its front page giving the impression new marijuana dangers had been uncovered. A more accurate conclusion from the article's data might be that psychiatric patients may turn to marijuana hoping to solve their problems. Too bad so many trees were sacrificed to print misleading noninformation.

Wiped Out

Dear Dr. Schoenfeld:

I've been smoking dope for about one year and have had many people tell me when you smoke you use up a lot of energy.

I think this is true because when I am low on energy and smoke some grass, I get really tired and wiped out. I don't think that it's because of the quality of the dope.

What's your side of the story?

ANSWER: Many people who formerly were heavy marijuana users have either given the drug up entirely or use it only now and then. They changed their habits because they didn't like the feeling of being continually wasted. Others go on periodic dope fasts for various lengths of time. Still others have used marijuana daily for years with no apparent change in their normal (or abnormal) functions.

Fatigue after using marijuana depends upon individual response as well as the quality of the grass. If marijuana wipes you out and you don't want to be wiped out—don't use it.

The federal government sponsors about 50 marijuana research projects. In order to supply these projects, the government entered into the following contracts: three contracts to produce synthetic THC (tetrahydrocannabinol), two contracts to test THC production methods, one to determine which components of marijuana smoke enter the user's system, and a contract to the University of Mississippi to grow five varieties of weed on ten acres of top-secret land. Let's see now . . . Gulfport Gold, Biloxi Boo, Anslinger Red. . . .

Dope for Senior Citizens?

Dear Dr. Schoenfeld:

I am 62 and retired by necessity (and how). Well, in the first place I have an incurable heart disease or rather two of them (infarctions and arteriosclerosis) plus high blood pressure. Also assorted other conditions.

The big trouble is that I have an anxiety neurosis, so I never know whether any symptom is physical or not. I have been like that since I was about 16. Though they really did try, I have wasted a small fortune on psychiatrists without any results whatsoever.

Tranquilizers make me sleepy and depressed or fearfully nervous after the effects have worn off. Alcohol simply makes me feel sick. Now marijuana, on the few happy occasions I have had an opportunity to smoke it, has made me calm, relaxed and happy and seems to leave no aftereffect. My great difficulty is contacting a reliable dealer since I cannot get around too much and my age would be against me also. How I wish I could!

I seem to have read somewhere that tests were being made with tetrahydrocannabinol (THC), the active principle of marijuana. Now I know that drug companies give samples of new drugs to physicians for clinical testing under field conditions and I wonder whether THC has arrived at that stage yet. For that matter, I would buy it on the black market if it were the genuine stuff. Do you happen to know any physician who would like a subject to test it on?

P.S. I am very careful about the use of all *drugs. Marijuana did not seem to affect my heart or blood pressure at all.*

ANSWER: No drug company has yet been authorized to conduct clinical trials with marijuana but the increasing illegal use of this drug by many segments of the population, old and young, rich and poor, will undoubtedly lead to widespread legal experiments.

THC Fraud

Dear Dr. Schoenfeld:

I am a 17-year-old boy living with my parents in a small town. I have been hearing and reading quite a bit about THC.

It would be a boon to us small-towners who want to turn on but are missed by any drug traffic.

Where can I get some THC?

ANSWER: THC, or tetrahydrocannabinol, is thought to be the active ingredient of marijuana. Because the synthesis of this drug is so complicated and expensive, any "THC" sold on the black market is almost surely not synthetic marijuana.

When samples of street "THC" are collected and analyzed, the capsules invariably are found to contain not THC, but PCP, a sedative used for treating animals.

Most dealers know little about the purity of the drugs they sell. The most widely known underground (al)chemist believes that a dealer with any feelings at all for other people will use the drug on himself first before selling it to others. Anyone selling you THC at this time is either ripping you off or doesn't know his hash from his elbow.

Marijuana and Childbirth

Dear Dr. Schoenfeld:

I am expecting my baby in about 4 weeks. In the past I have read many articles on marijuana stating that long ago it was used for medical purposes.

I wonder if marijuana would be useful during childbirth. I know it would relax you, but do you think it would also decrease the labor pains and bring on delivery faster?

It is a shame the research on marijuana isn't being done

on all its aspects. They may find some remarkably good benefits. If it did help during labor it would be a wonderful thing.

ANSWER: One important reason for practicing natural childbirth is that the baby is born free of drugs which might otherwise be given the mother. Marijuana used during labor might adversely affect the baby's ability to breathe.

Brought Down by Tobacco

Dear Dr. Schoenfeld:

I've been smoking grass for one meager year and tobacco for one meager month. Since I've started cigarettes, I've been unable to attain any sort of respectable high.

Do you think stopping tobacco would help?

ANSWER: Maybe, maybe not. But the practice of smoking cigarettes is a known health hazard leading to lung cancer, emphysema and possibily peptic ulcers and heart disease.

Dangerous Hobbies

Dear Dr. Hip:

I recently read an interesting article about the art of growing marijuana. This seems like an interesting and pleasurable hobby for a harassed physician in Oklahoma.

I had to give up one of my hobbies as automobile drivers have become very aggressive toward motorcycle riders on anything larger than a Honda 80. This leaves me with only my Sunday School class.

Please advise me whether it would be better to be busted for pot or busted up on my cycle.

ANSWER: Whichever hobby you decide to pursue, you'd better wear a helmet for safety.

Horny Heads

Dear Dr. Schoenfeld:

I have noticed that guys stoned on grass are usually horny, but girls aren't. Any comments?

ANSWER: Maybe their horns don't show.

To Tell the Truth

Early one morning I received a telephone call from a lady with Goodson-Todman Enterprises Limited. Would I like to appear on the newly resuscitated "To Tell The Truth" program? To tell the truth I wanted to go to New York anyway so I agreed.

Backstage at the Ed Sullivan Theater were a parade of Hawaiian dancers, Mandarin singers, foppish clothes designers, three Mrs. Joe Garagiolas and the Drs. Schoenfeld. The other Drs. Schoenfeld were a short-haired stockbroker and a bearded newscaster from Hackensack.

After the real me stood up I was asked medical questions by the studio audience.

Their questions were similar to those I had been answering in my column, mostly about sex and drugs. A lady asked about blood clots and birth control pills. I said several studies of large-dose birth control pills indicated that women who took the "pill" had, statistically, a greater chance of developing blood clots than those who did not use them. But the dangers to a normal woman during pregnancy are still greater than if she takes birth control pills.

An elderly man asked about sex education for children. My answer was that I thought a child's questions should all be answered to the limits of his ability to understand, whatever his age.

A young fellow asked if I thought marijuana should be legalized. My reply was something like, "So far as scientists know, alcohol is more harmful than marijuana. I think marijuana should be subject to the same regulations."

But the marijuana question is not so simple that it can be dismissed in two sentences on a daytime quiz show.

What does legalization of marijuana mean? The relatively low-potency marijuana leaf used by most pot heads today? Hashish? Tetrahydrocannabinol, marijuana's active ingredient, which can cause a full-blown psychedelic trip when taken in sufficient quantities?

Would "legalization" of marijuana lead to a decrease in

the number of alcoholics? How many skid row marijuana bums could we expect?

Among the unanswered questions are the actual numbers of American marijuana users. The United States Department of Health, Education and Welfare estimates 24 million and this seems a conservative figure. Certainly the use of grass in large cities and on college campuses must remind some graybeards of the days of alcohol prohibition.

Why has the use of marijuana become so widespread? Fad? Maybe. But its use continues to grow. A better high than alcohol without a hangover? You bet, heads will say. But many people prefer alcohol even when marijuana is freely available. A symbol of rebellion? Perhaps to some. But many political militants condemn the use of drugs as counterrevolutionary. A communist plot, as the wife of a college dean once asked me? The Russians have their own problems with drug users. An aphrodisiac? Marijuana seems to enhance or intensify sexual feelings if people are turned on to each other in the first place. But if they are turned off to each other, marijuana intensifies the turnoff.

Whatever the reasons, the United States government believes there are over 24 million Americans whose use of this drug subjects them to penalties. Our jails are schools for crime. Compulsory drug clinics allow marijuana users to learn about narcotics directly from addicts.

Marijuana is neither a noxious weed nor a harmless flower. Most people find its effects beneficial or merely enjoyable when used in moderation. Others receive no effect from the drug, bum out or, in rare cases, become temporarily psychotic. But so far as I can determine, the most harmful known aspect of marijuana use in normal mature individuals is the possibility of arrest and imprisonment.

LSD

. . . When the LSD started to work, I was in my home with my wife. She shrank, and she became very small. It is a very funny experience, but it is difficult to explain LSD. It is not the same feeling that comes after too many drinks or taking sedatives. It is the opposite. The brain nerves or brain cells are affected, they become sharper. It is as though I stood next to myself, and while these hallucinations take place I know all the time this is not reality. It was a very strange, amusing and central feeling to touch my skin. I still remember very clearly I had a more sensual feeling than I ever had before simply touching my hands one with the other. It's an amazing experience and I'm glad I did it. . . .

Otto Preminger
p. 162, *The Cinema of Otto Preminger*
by Gerald Pratley, A. S. Barnes & Co.,
New York, 1971

Dear Dr. Schoenfeld:

Three and a half years ago I took some LSD. A good trip ensued. Insights into my place in nature were gained and no monstrous obsessions surfaced. Nevertheless, I haven't had any since, never having felt the desire or need to.

Last July I impregnated my wife. The thought that I may have unwittingly fathered a monster is destroying my peace. I'm afraid to talk about it with my wife as I don't want to worry her unless necessary.

So what are the chances that the LSD trip could've

altered my chromosomes? Can I have this checked? Where? How? Should we consider terminating the pregnancy?

ANSWER: Distortion of "reality" is an effect attributed to the psychedelic drug LSD. But more dangerous distortions may be caused by those who oppose new ideas out of fear, ignorance and prejudice. The psychedelic drug controversy may well be remembered in history as ranking with the persecution of those who thought the earth was round or doubted that the universe moved about the earth.

How did the LSD-chromosome story begin? One day a physician visiting the San Francisco area for a medical meeting was walking through the Haight-Ashbury district at the height of the "flower children" era. He gawked at hippies in beads, long hair and flowers, shook his head and said, "My God, look at those kids. Something must be wrong with their chromosomes." Then (contrary to the rules of scientific procedure) he set out to prove that LSD was harmful.

Shortly afterward, several reports purported to prove that LSD was harmful to chromosomes and each was widely reported in newspapers and magazines. But scientific investigations and conclusions require time. Only now is a balanced picture of the chromosome question emerging.

In the October 27, 1967, *Science*, a team of researchers from the Lawrence Radiation Laboratory of the University of California at Berkeley, reported their study of chromosomes of LSD users and nonusers. The same results were found in an unpublished study by Dr. Nicolas Petrakis, a hematologist of the University of California School of Medicine at San Francisco. These two studies finding no chromosomal damage in LSD users received little notice.

Child psychiatrists Bender and Sankar of the Creedmoor State Hospital in New York were disturbed by reports of LSD-induced chromosomal damage because they had treated schizophrenic children with pure known LSD in quantities of 100 to 150 micrograms every day for from 5½ to 35 months. The children's chromosomes were examined 20 to 48 months after LSD therapy ended and were found to be unchanged. Bender and Sankar's findings were reported in the February 16, 1968, *Science*.

A series of one does not make a scientific study but it is of interest to note that Timothy Leary, who has taken LSD well over 1000 times, had his chromosomes examined through Harvard University's Medical School. They were found to be normal.

An article in the November 3, 1969, *Journal of the A.M.A.* reported no alteration in the chromosomes of 32 patients participating in an LSD study sponsored by Baltimore's Spring Grove State Hospital and the National Institute for Mental Health.

A review of published studies of LSD in the April 30, 1971, *Science* by Dishotsky, Loughman, Mogar and Lipscomb concludes that LSD does not damage chromosomes, has never been proven to cause birth defects (but like any other drug should not be used during pregnancy), and does not produce cancer. The authors conclude that "other than during pregnancy, there is no present contraindication to the continued controlled experimental use of pure LSD."

Apparently, the government supports researchers who desperately seek damaging effects from LSD. The latest pseudoscientific LSD study comes from the University of Illinois at Urbana. Edward W. Voss, Jr., and his associates reported LSD inhibited formation of antibodies, which the body needs to fight disease. Much newspaper coverage for these "revelations." But the fine print tells us that even if we weren't reading about test tube experiments, a human would have to ingest thousands of times the usual LSD dose to produce the same results. Reports like these make scientists look stupid in the eyes of young people. And rightly so. There are enough real dangers of improper LSD use without the addition of counterproductive scare tactics.

LSD Freakouts

A report in the July 15, 1968, *Journal of the A.M.A.* indicates that psychotic reactions following LSD use may occur most often in those with a previous history of psychiatric illness and hospitalization.

The authors, Drs. Hekimian and Gershon, psychiatrists with the N.Y.U. School of Medicine, studied one out of five patients admitted to Bellevue Psychiatric Hospital over a six-month period in 1967. Speaking of the psychedelic group of patients they say, "A striking feature, as with the marijuana and amphetamine groups, was the high percentage of preexisting schizophrenia."

The authors then ask, "Are prolonged adverse psychotic reactions to the psychedelic drugs due to the drug per se, or are they in fact often due to the preexisting psychiatric illness?"

Many investigators have noted that a large proportion of individuals with psychiatric illness use drugs like LSD in an attempt at self-medication. Those who suffer adverse and prolonged reactions following LSD use undoubtedly reflect this highly skewed population.

Dear Dr. Schoenfeld:

While my daughter was in college she took LSD 14 times and Methedrine intravenously, 2 grams weekly, average dose.

She is now 23 and has paranoid schizophrenia. (It's been 2 years since it was diagnosed.)

I can't seem to get a straight answer from anyone anywhere, so I'm writing to you in hopes you can tell me:

1. *Could her psychosis have been directly drug induced?*
2. *It appears she probably had an hereditary predisposition to schizophrenia, although her behavior and perception were essentially normal until she was 19 and started taking the drugs.*

   If she did indeed have this predisposition, would it have evolved during her college years anyway, drug ingestion or not?
3. *Or, had she not taken the drugs, would it have remained in its initial, latent phase?*

4. *If, indeed, the drugs were a contributing factor, which one was it—LSD or Speed or both?*

I would certainly appreciate any straight information you could give me.

ANSWER: Many people with psychiatric ailments use drugs in a conscious or unconscious attempt at self-treatment. There's no way of knowing whether or not your daughter would have manifested her schizophrenia without the use of LSD and Methedrine (methamphetamine). Some patients who require long-term hospitalization after drug-induced experiences have no prior history of psychiatric problems—but most do.

In short, there's no way of really answering your questions except to guess—and my guess might be different from someone else's guess.

One thing is certain though, people predisposed to psychiatric illness run an added risk when they use drugs without medical supervision.

LSD Flashbacks

One of the many unanswered questions about LSD concerns flashbacks—unexpected recurrences of the psychedelic trip long after the drug has left the body. Most people experiencing flashbacks find them very unpleasant experiences.

Since use of LSD is illegal we have no idea of the true incidence of flashbacks. The great majority of those who use mind-altering drugs never come to the attention of health personnel, educators or the police.

Impure drugs, unstable individuals, frequent trips and, most importantly, psychological stress may be factors contributing to acid flashbacks. On the other hand all these factors may be found in the case of a person who has never had flashbacks. Mardi Horowitz, M.D., a research psychiatrist at San Francisco's Mt. Zion Hospital postulates several theories explaining flashbacks in *Image Formation and Cognition*, Appleton-Century Crofts, New York, 1970.

1. *The Release Theory:* Repeated use of LSD may produce long-lasting changes in neurophysiologic brain processes inhibiting image formation.
2. *Deconditioning Theory:* The LSD experience produces a heightened awareness of images. Ordinarily we suppress certain images in order to function more effectively in what we usually consider reality. Once another reality is experienced some individuals may not return completely to their original state.
3. *Psychodynamic Theory:* Concern with the inner world, rejection of the external world including other persons, and an intrinsic interest in imagery combine to produce flashbacks in members of the "drug community."
4. *The Mystic Theory:* The brain contains imprinted memories of past ages. Once brought to consciousness through psychedelics the images return over and over again.

Dear Dr. Schoenfeld:

Ever since I took acid (about 6 months ago) I still see things after I come down. There's a negative of everything when I close my eyes and tracers of everything. Not as intense as when I'm on the drug but they are there.

Don't get me wrong, I really like the stuff. What I want to know is will this ever stop and is it safe to take acid or mescaline again?

P.S. I've taken acid 6 times.

Dear Dr. Hip Pocrates:

I am a sixteen-year-old girl. I have dropped acid around 60–70 times but stopped dropping it around 6 months ago (except for 2 times three months ago).

Well, I am permanently hallucinating, like seeing the walls moving and flashing colors and lights. It bothers me that I still hallucinate as much as I did months ago.

I've heard of flashbacks but I'm always seeing these things. Do you know why this is?

ANSWER: The true incidence of flashbacks is unknown but they are frequently reported as a side effect of LSD use. Usually flashbacks are unwanted and disturbing experiences.

Tranquilizers and a limited period of counseling or psychotherapy are usually sufficient to treat LSD flashbacks.

Both of you live near free medical clinics where you can be treated with a minimum of hassle.

Brain Damage?

Dear Dr. Hip Pocrates:

Is it possible that one's brain could be damaged by a bad trip on LSD? If so, what can be done about this?

Since the bad trip about a month ago, I feel strange and just on the verge of tripping most of the time. Objects appear to be deformed and different from what I remember them to be before the bad trip. This frightens me and keeps me continually nervous and on edge.

I don't have the money to go to a doctor or psychiatrist, so what can I do?

ANSWER: You may be eligible for free medical care through your local welfare department. Call them to find out. There's also a free clinic in your city which treats drug problems similar to the one you describe.

Pure LSD is not known to cause brain damage but when buying drugs on the street you can't be certain of the drug you're getting.

Strychnine in LSD

WARNING: Analysis of street LSD samples has at times indicated the addition of strychnine. The drug is apparently added to LSD because of its stimulatory effects on the spinal cord. No longer used in medicine, strychnine is sold commerically as a rat poison.

Some people risk high doses of LSD because they know its toxicity in man is very low. Should the tabs or capsules contain strychnine they might die like a rat. Symptoms are similar to tetanus poisoning—massive muscle spasms, extreme sensitivity to light, sound or touch. Death results from suffocation or exhaustion after a prolonged series of painful convulsions.

After Many a Summer

Dear Dr. Schoenfeld:

How did Aldous Huxley die? I've heard rumors that he took a massive overdose of LSD because he wanted to experience death. Is that true?

ANSWER: No known human death has ever occurred as the result of an LSD overdose. I'm speaking of pure, not adulterated, LSD. And I'm not including suicides or accidental deaths.

Aldous Huxley died of cancer on November 22, 1963. His early experiences with mescaline were described in *The Doors of Perception*, published in 1954.

Several medical studies have indicated LSD relieves suffering and fear in people facing imminent death. The insight gained into life processes allowed them to accept death more peacefully. Aldous Huxley is said to have taken LSD just before he died.

LSD and Ergot

Dear Dr. Schoenfeld:

On an acid trip I took recently, my left hand and arm went totally dead on me. This has happened twice before on very heavy acid trips. I have taken acid about 60 times in the last three years.

Anyway, like I said, my left arm went dead. I couldn't move it very well and I could barely make a fist of my fingers. In about 3 hours my left hand and arm were back to normal use but I was worried by the incident. Oh, by the way, it has always been my left hand and arm that have gone dead.

Is this a normal occurrence or is something wrong? I haven't taken any acid trips lately nor do I plan to until I find out about this.

ANSWER: All "LSD" available on the black market today is illegally produced by chemists who, of necessity, run makeshift laboratories. Compounds produced in these laboratories contain impurities which may be more dangerous than the pure drugs.

LSD is related to ergot, a substance which causes constriction of blood vessels including those in the brain. Ergot is a fungus which grows on rye and other grains. During the Middle Ages epidemics of ergot poisoning occurred in which the characteristic symptoms were gangrene of the feet, legs, hands and arms.

If I were you I would have a thorough physical examination. You may have taken an impure drug or you might have a medical condition causing the symptoms you describe.

Fasting and LSD

Dear Dr. Hip Pocrates:

I am going on a fast for 4–5 days at the end of which I plan to drop some acid. Will there be any added risks or more physiological problems beyond those when taking acid when well nourished? I am taking vitamins.

ANSWER: Even under the most favorable circumstances an LSD experience is physically wearing. A four or five day fast will leave you in a weakened condition and physical harm might then result from taking LSD.

Mixed Emotions?

Dear Dr. Schoenfeld:

Both myself and my wife live a day-to-day tragedy in the form of my mother-in-law's mental condition. She lays in bed all day long, does not clean the house, has tried to commit suicide, and refuses to voluntarily sign herself into a mental facility. In short, she does not have any will left to live, and she is only 48 years old. She only says she wants to die.

Then yesterday I had an idea to change her state of mind (it couldn't get any worse) and let her go on some trips with some super LSD. I have had a lot of experience on acid although I haven't taken any for the last 1½ years. I feel confident that a few good trips and I could instill the will in her that she so desperately needs to go on. She has consented to take the acid.

The main question we would like to know is if you feel this would be a constructive measure, and if so, should we have some Thorazine on hand just in case she freaks out. We also wondered if there is any possible danger from LSD in a person so disoriented as she.

ANSWER: The people most likely to do poorly under the influence of LSD are those with a previous history of serious psychiatric illness. Although you might wish nothing but good for your mother-in-law, the results could prove to be disastrous.

Ironic, isn't it, that you or any other lay person can buy all the LSD you wish in any city or on any college campus, while physicians are forbidden by the government to use LSD or other mind-expanding drugs in treating their patients.

Since your mother-in-law agreed to take LSD perhaps she would accept other treatment methods. She might also be eligible for regular visits from a nurse through the Visiting Nurse Association. Call them or your local health department for further information.

Electric Kool-Aid

During a chartered plane flight, I watched someone walking up the aisle asking for contributions to a psychedelic punch. Some people threw in drugs *said to be* LSD and mescaline. I emphasize "said to be" because most black market drugs turn out to be something else either in quality or composition. The drugs were mixed with a punch and the bowl passed around. Most people used their heads and abstained.

Drinking from such an electric punch is like playing Russian roulette with your brain cells. Even if drugs are pure they may interact badly with each other, to say nothing of the unknown strength of the punch or the wisdom of using drugs in those circumstances.

I've also seen electric punch bowls at parties, usually, but not always, labeled as such. The punch may become available to children if they are present, just as many kids surreptitiously sip the remains of alcoholic drinks when their parents aren't looking.

Accidental Ingestion in a Baby

Dear Dr. Schoenfeld:

Recently my 14-month-old daughter got a hold of some LSD tabs. The trip was apparently too much for her because she kept crying out in what seemed to be terror.

My husband sat with her for the most part because I fell apart seeing her like that. In the end, the acid did wear off and she slept that night and a good part of the next day.

Since then she seems to be back to the way she was before. She didn't flip out for good and yet she is not the youngest "enlightened one" on earth. She is just a little girl baby.

The reason I am writing: I expect this same thing has happened and will happen to others. I think it would be valuable for any parent to know how to handle a stoned child. I would suggest also that the mother take a good strong tranquilizer so as to make matters as calm as possible.

ANSWER: Accidents and poisonings are, by far, the greatest killers of children in the United States. About 400 children between 1 and 4 years of age die each year in this country because parents leave drugs or chemicals within their reach.

Substances which most frequently cause dangerous poisoning are listed as follows in Dr. Ben Spock's *Baby and Child Care* (a book every mother should own—Pocket Books, 95¢):

Aspirin and other drugs
Insect and rat poisons
Kerosene, gasoline, benzene and cleaning fluids
Lead in paint that a child has chewed off something

(Most indoor paint and toy paint contain no lead. The danger is from outdoor paint on windowsills, porches, etc., and from outdoor paint that has been used at home to repaint toys, cribs and other furniture.)

Liquid furniture and auto polish

Lye, alkalis used for cleaning drains, bowls, ovens

Oil of wintergreen

Plant sprays.

LSD tabs or caps have been shown to contain highly toxic substances such as strychnine or belladonna. A "stoned" child should receive immediate medical care.

At present, free clinics know best how to handle this kind of accident. Some people with drug problems won't go to a general hospital for fear they'll be turned in to the police. If people avoid medical care for this reason, the hospital is acting against the public interest.

Be sure to tell your pediatrician or family physician about this accident. But don't become overprotective toward your little girl. She'll most likely be completely normal—if you keep dangerous substances where she can't get at them.

What?

Dear Dr. Schoenfeld:

Do LSD or other psychedelics cause memory loss?

ANSWER: I can't remember reading any such report.

Peyote and Mescaline

Peyote (*Lophophora williamsii*) is a small, spineless cactus with a gray-green top or "button" and a brown carrot-shaped root. The part of the plant extending above the ground is cut off and usually dried to form the peyote "button."

Some evidence indicates Mexican Indians used the plant for ceremonial purposes as early as 300 B.C. Spanish conquistadors described its use as early as 1560. The Spanish invaders denounced peyote as a diabolical root and in 1620 passed a law against its use:

"We the Inquisitors against heretical perversity and apostasy, by virtue of apostolic authority declare . . . it is an act of superstition: condemned—as opposed to the purity and integrity of our Holy Catholic Faith. The fantasies suggest intervention of the devil; the real authority of this vice."

Peyote use probably spread to Texas around 1870 though it may have occurred in that region earlier. The plant was used seasonally in Mexico but throughout the year amongst the Plains Indians of the United States. Christian elements were gradually added to the peyote ceremony, and in 1914 the "First-born Church of Christ" was organized. This was later to become the "Native American Church" which now claims more than 200,000 members. Peyotism is the native religion of more than 50 American tribes including the Cheyenne, Arapaho, Chippewa, Blackfoot, Crow, Delaware, Shawnee, Pawnee and Sioux.

The December, 1972, *National Geographic* quotes a Native American Church member who felt ritual use of peyote had benefited him and his family:

"My family has used peyote since 1959. Until then we only had a hogan. Now we live in a house. We sleep on beds instead of sheepskins. Now my parents don't fight. I have a job and a pickup."

According to the article, most of the 40,000 Navajos belonging to the Church also believe the peyote rites have improved their lives.

The peyote cactus contains nine interactive alkaloids which together are known as peyotl (or panpeyotl). Mescaline is the most active component but psychedelic connoisseurs consistently claim subtle differences exist between peyote and mescaline.

Mescaline was isolated from peyote in 1896 and chemically synthesized in 1919. The drug was used by such respected nineteenth-century scientists as William James and Havelock Ellis. Ellis found the experience "an educational influence of no mean value."

Peyote and mescaline often cause nausea and vomiting—otherwise the immediate physiological effects are minimal. There has never been a long-term study of the effects of mescaline or peyote on humans.

One of the "accusations" made against peyote is that the drug is an aphrodisiac. According to psychologist William H. McGlothlin, "the only persons who find peyote to be a reliable aphrodisiac are missionaries and magazine writers." And at least one medical columnist.

Most states permit use of peyote by bona fide members of the Native American Church. Mescaline use is prohibited by federal law except for selected research groups. The effects of both drugs last approximately 10–12 hours and wear off gradually. Bad trips are possible but seem to be rare. In 1971, a U.S. Public Health Service physician who had worked with members of the Native American Church estimated bad peyote trips occurred 1 in 70,000 times.

A fascinating account of a Native American Church ceremony by Stewart Brand, founder of the *Whole Earth Catalog*, was published in an issue of *Psychedelic Review*.

Quanan Parker, an early peyote leader, said, "The white man goes into his church house and talks *about* Jesus; the Indian goes into his tepee and talks *to* Jesus."

Mescaline Fantasies

Dear Dr. Hip:

I have heard various stories regarding mescaline and peyote use, the most prevalent being that it absorbs your bone marrow.

Is this a fact or a fallacy?

ANSWER: A fantasy. Any psychedelic may precipitate a bad trip (such as imagining your bone marrow is being absorbed) but physical harm has not been reported from these drugs.

Believing you have mescaline may itself be a fantasy since recent analyses of street drugs have shown the "mescaline" is usually an entirely different drug—such as STP or LSD.

Dear Dr. Schoenfeld:

I was told recently by a pharmacist that mescaline was an alkaloid and therefore was harmful to the human body. In fact, he said it was the most harmful of the drugs now popular and that in the human male attacked the testicles. Help!

ANSWER: Most psychedelic drugs are alkaloids, including mescaline. Although any psychedelic drug can cause a bad trip, mescaline seems to cause fewer bad experiences than LSD. Most drug samples sold as mescaline in the street turn out to be STP, LSD or some other drug. Mescaline does often seem to go right to the testicles but the drug affects all the other senses as well. There is no evidence whatsoever that pure mescaline physically damages the testicles or other parts of the body.

The most harmful of the drugs now popular is alcohol.

Dear Dr. Schoenfeld:

Speaking of the agony and the ecstasy, are you aware of any possible connection between recurrent bladder infections and mescaline?

ANSWER: No. But bladder infections (and diseases in general) are often linked to one's emotional state.

Flashbacks Revisited

Dear Dr. Schoenfeld:

Does mescaline cause flashbacks as LSD can?

ANSWER: Flashbacks from any psychedelic are theoretically possible but no verified cases have been reported for pure mescaline. Even those who have obtained real mescaline have usually used LSD sometime in the past.

Street Drug Analysis

Dr. Schoenfeld:

In a recent column you commented that it would be unusual to find real mescaline on the black market. It has been my contention right along that there is none to be had. The same with THC, synthetic or organic (which is also a big shuck for the most part). I also believe that all LSD on the black market contains many impurities which are often mistaken for speed.

ANSWER: Investigators at the New Jersey Neuro-Psychiatric Institute obtained and analyzed 36 samples from users. Most, but not all, of the samples said to be LSD were really LSD (though the amounts of LSD ranged from 50 to 283 micrograms). NONE of the drugs sold as mescaline, psilocybin or THC (tetrahydrocannabinol) turned out to be those substances. Four samples of alleged mescaline were actually STP.

Similar findings are reported weekly by the Los Angeles Do It Now Foundation and Palo Alto's Pharm Chem Laboratories. However the drugs are packaged—tablets or capsules of various sizes or colors—rarely, if ever, is any mescaline found on the street. Instead, LSD or LSD-PCP combinations are pushed as mescaline or psilocybin to gullible consumers.

During Pregnancy

Dear Dr. Schoenfeld:

Do you offer any precautions against taking mescaline during childbirth? It seems ideal for maximum mental alertness and physical endurance.

If the idea is a very dangerous one, perhaps you can suggest a similar, safer drug. But I'd really like to try it for those reasons.

ANSWER: One of the great failings of our educational system is that students can go through grade school and college and never study the human body. Students taking a course in human physiology would learn that an unborn baby's circulation is linked to the mother's—drugs taken by the mother also affect the child. Physicians administer drugs during childbirth with great care because of possible effects on the fetus.

The best way to insure the health of your unborn child is to eat a nutritious diet, abstain from all drugs (including alcohol and tobacco) and receive regular examinations from your family physician or obstetrician.

Dear Dr. Schoenfeld:

Is there a danger in taking MDA, psilocybin or mescaline during pregnancy? Because these are chemicals, I wonder if they are harmful to the baby?

ANSWER: Yes, yes, yes to your questions. Do not take those or any other drugs during pregnancy lest they deform or kill your unborn baby. Even cigarette smoking is known to increase sterility, cause babies to have lower birth weights and increase the numbers of stillbirths.

Dear Dr. Schoenfeld:

I am pregnant and do not intend to take any trips during the first three months. My friends say after that organic psilocybin would not be harmful. Is this so?

How are trips on a natural substance different from synthetics?

ANSWER: Your friends may mean well but they are not giving you good advice. It's true that the first three months (first trimester) of pregnancy is the most critical time in the development of the fetus. But some substances can cause changes even late in pregnancy. Tetracycline, for example, taken by the expectant mother in the second or third trimester can cause changes in the bones and teeth of her unborn child. You should not take psilocybin or any other drug while you are carrying your child.

I assume that by "organic" psilocybin you refer to an actual extract from Mexican "magic" mushrooms rather than a compound synthesized in a laboratory. Unless you have actually seen these chemicals being produced you have no way of knowing whether they are "organic" or synthetic or even the drug they are said to be. Moreover, there is no reason to believe that extracted chemicals cause different trips from those entirely synthesized. There are subtle differences between the trips caused by peyote and mescaline and between psilocybin and magic mushrooms. But the "organic" vs. synthetic question is just a shuck used to sell drugs, comparable to Madison Avenue gimmicks. Incidentally, psilocybin was first produced in the laboratory in 1958 by A. Hoffman, the same Swiss chemist who initially synthesized LSD.

Dear Doctor:

I have two very important questions that I need any *and* immediate *information on.*

I am somewhere between 2 and 3 mos. pregnant with a baby that I want very much to have. For the following reasons, however, I'm considering applying for a therapeutic abortion if there are any doubts as to the effect on the fetus of the following:

(1) *I have just come down with hepatitis (most likely serum type).*

(2) *Last month, before I knew I was pregnant I took what is passing for THC on the streets, maybe about 7 or 8 caps at different times. I just read one of those scare articles that talked of "deformed babies from what was probably the street THC."*

Please send me anything you know about both hepatitis and this THC. And please, as soon as possible.

ANSWER: If you have just come down with hepatitis your doctor has probably already told you this is not an indication for a therapeutic abortion. The magazine article is correct in that what is passing for THC is not that drug at all. But no one really knows how harmful this fake THC is to unborn children. If you want to have a baby the chances are it would be born perfectly normal, though of course deformities may occur even when no drugs are taken during pregnancy. In any case, you should now be under the care of a physician who can care for you during your pregnancy.

STP Drops Four-Year-Old

The largest known human dose of STP was ingested accidentally by a four-year-old boy in Southern California. His parents returned home to find as many as 40 STP tablets missing and the child lying on the floor convulsing. For several hours they hesitated to take him to a hospital, hoping the seizures would stop, fearful they would be turned over to the police. When he finally reached a hospital, a partial paralysis existed on one side of his body. After two days he was able to respond to questions. The paralysis gradually subsided but he remained mute for a long time.

This unhappy incident is told to remind parents that small children are apt to pop medicine into their mouths if they can find it, especially brightly colored or candy-coated tablets or capsules. The most common household medicine, aspirin, kills more children each year than any other drug or poison.

Why should people have to fear that physicians might act as agents of the police? It's time that doctors began to act as independently in their primary role of treating patients as they are when dealing with economic matters.

Tobacco

The Real Killer Weed

One in every 40 deaths in the United States is caused by lung cancer, and this ratio is expected to increase in the next 10 years.

What has been the response of cigarette manufacturers? They've made their cigarettes longer, thereby hooking the user all the more.

Tobacco is an addicting drug. The more one smokes, the harder it is to give up the habit. Those extra little millimeters added to already king-size cancer sticks are more than a promotional gimmick.

Cigarettes and Pregnancy

The cause for most birth defects and miscarriages in this country is unknown. Cigarette smoking may be a major factor.

An article in the *Archives of Environmental Health* reported a study of 2016 married women which revealed that cigarette-smoking women had an increased rate of miscarriages, fewer pregnancies and more infertility.

Pipes and Cigars

People who have switched from cigarettes to pipes or cigars may only have traded lung cancer for kidney cancer.

Cancer of the kidney occurs five times as much in cigarette smokers as in those who do not use tobacco at all. But pipe and cigar smokers run twice the risk of cigarette smokers of developing cancer of the kidney, reported two Seattle pathologists in *Cancer*. Pipe and cigar smokers usually do not inhale so the site of irritation isn't the lungs. Instead, the smoke is absorbed by mucous membranes of the mouth or the stomach, circulated through the bloodstream and filtered by the kidneys.

Innocent Victims

Antibiotic News contained an interesting item about unwitting victims of tobacco freaks.

Dr. Paul Cameron, of Wayne State University, found that children of tobacco users have twice as much respiratory disease as children in nonsmoking families.

"We also were able to correlate the amount of sickness with the amount of smoke in the household. The more smoke, the more respiratory illness."

Dr. Cameron said that all the differences between the "smoke" and "no-smoke" groups were statistically significant.

"Children are known to be particularly susceptible to air pollution. And these findings, though not definitive, suggest that they are also particularly susceptible to that air pollution caused by cigarette, cigar and pipe smoke," the Wayne State physician concluded.

Withdrawal Symptoms

Dear Dr. Schoenfeld:

Heeding the Surgeon General's advice, I smoked my last cigarette a week ago. Now I find my body reacting in strange ways. For the past week I have been able to sleep at night at most only six hours while before I averaged well over 10 (unless disturbed). I wake up after six hours and cannot go back. Though I feel rested I wonder why I sleep less. Do you know?

In addition, I find that my ejaculations have undergone a fantastic reduction in intensity. Though my erections are healthy, my ejaculations are meager little squirts (the semen just oozes out), while previously they were powerful pumps. It feels as if my penis is clogged or my supply of semen is lacking. I've tried waiting two days without intercourse with no effect. Would smoking relieve this condition? What do you recommend?

ANSWER: Camels, if the symptoms you described were directly related to cessation of cigarette smoking. But, so far as I know, these symptoms are not related to cigarette smoking or the stopping of cigarette smoking. The time required for kicking the cigarette habit varies greatly but you might notice changes in your sleeping habits for a month or two afterward. You will soon notice your senses of taste, hearing and smell have become keener and I would suspect that you would become more powerful in all ways within a few months.

Effect on Blood

Blood from donors who smoke is probably less useful therapeutically than that from nonsmokers. Investigators of the University of Florida College of Medicine have found that toxic agents in tobacco smoke, especially cigarettes, cause the body to generate a substance which greatly reduces oxygen transport by red blood cells. Reduced oxygen transport may contribute to heart attacks. Robert Elliot, M.D., who led the investigations, said, "These changes are apparent even in a young person who smokes more than 12 cigarettes a day."

A report in the *Journal of the A.M.A.* of March 30, 1970, indicates smokers not only have 11 times more lung cancer than nonsmokers, but that heavy smokers develop a more malignant form of the disease than the lung cancer seen in light smokers.

Tobacco Pushers Want Nicotine

On a visit to Bavaria I met a German inventor who had patented a method of removing nicotine from tobacco. He couldn't find one manufacturer interested in the process. Why? Nicotine apparently is important in the process which causes addiction to cigarettes and the tobacco industry wants to keep its customers hooked.

Filters on cigarettes may turn out to be nothing but a gimmick. A study in the *British Medical Journal* of September 19, 1970, reported observations on 36 cigarette smokers. Some used "high retention" filters and some "low retention" filters. Those using "high retention" filters puffed their cigarettes more frequently and thus received nearly the same amount of nicotine as those using "low retention" filters.

Amphetamines

Borrowed Speed

Dear Dr. Schoenfeld:

I've just started my freshman year in college and due to the starchy food in the dormitory cafeteria have gained 7 lbs. My roommate has some diet pills prescribed by her doctor. How many should I take? Is there any danger?

ANSWER: It's almost always dangerous to take a prescription medication without supervision from a physician. Otherwise all drugs could be purchased freely at pharmacy counters.

Many different kinds of "diet pills" are used to help control the appetite. The most commonly prescribed for this purpose are the amphetamines—dextroamphetamine (Dexedrine), methamphetamine (Desoxyn, Methedrine) and amphetamine (Benzedrine). The usual dose is 5–10 milligrams by mouth three times a day. Some drug companies package longer-acting preparations which may be taken only once a day.

When used properly and for short periods of time, diet pills can aid dieting by curbing the appetite. But all too frequently they are misused. Tolerance (the necessity to take more and more of a drug to achieve the same results) develops quickly with amphetamines. I have seen housewives who started out taking diet pills as directed and wound up gulping 100 of them each day.

Two effects of amphetamines, besides suppressing appetite, are to elevate the mood and postpone fatigue. Speed freaks abuse their bodies by ingesting large quantities of the drug, sniffing it or shooting it into their veins. But due to the phenomenon of tolerance more and more of the drug is used. Meth heads commonly shoot 100 to 300 milligrams of "crystals" every few hours when on a "run," amounts which could be immediately fatal for someone who had not developed tolerance.

Toxic psychoses and personality changes may result from long-term abuse of amphetamines. In short, amphetamines are valuable drugs when used properly but can be quite dangerous if misused.

When trying to lose weight, keep in mind that you must take in fewer calories than you expend. Try cutting down or eliminating potatoes, pastries, cakes, pies, candy, bread, soft drinks, pizza and beer. Your doctor can help you begin an organized diet.

Daily exercise is important but choose one that will fit easily into your life, otherwise you'll soon drop it.

Exams and Amphetamines

Dear Dr. Schoenfeld:

What is the danger of taking successive amphetamines to stay speedy while studying?

ANSWER: Amphetamines rapidly produce "tolerance," the pharmacologic phenomenon of needing to take more and more of the drug to achieve the same desired effect. When the effect of amphetamines wears off, depression follows, so some people keep taking more speed to avoid this unpleasant feeling. Soon they may become strung out on the drug. Toxic paranoid psychoses, overdoses, malnutrition, tooth decay and personality changes all may result from a chronic amphetamine habit.

Chest Pain

Dear Dr. Schoenfeld:

I have been taking certain types of speed, notably methamphetamine (Methedrine) and amphetamine (Benzedrine).

Along with the obvious appetite loss and sleep loss, I have experienced a dull pain that seems to come from beneath my sternum [breastbone].

This only appears while the speed is in effect. Maybe you could give me some advice about this.

ANSWER: If you have not had a medical examination recently, you should have one soon. One of the effects of amphetamines is to increase heart rate and blood pressure. The pain you feel while on amphetamines may very well be coming from your heart.

Small Doses Harmful?

Dear Dr. Schoenfeld:

According to a recent article, doctors have discovered that chronic intravenous use of speed can cause fatal degeneration of the capillaries.

My question: does speed in pill form have the same

effect? I nervously await your answer as I've become accustomed to taking a 15 mgm amphetamine capsule (prescribed) several times weekly to channel my energies for painting.

ANSWER: The article in question reported a fatal disease of blood vessels among abusers of multiple drugs. Intravenous methamphetamine (Methedrine) was suspected but not proven to be the causative agent.

No evidence exists to indicate that use of amphetamine in oral form in the dose you describe leads to physical or mental harm in healthy individuals. Amphetamines and amphetaminelike drugs (Ritalin, e.g.) are administered daily for "hyperactive" schoolchildren otherwise unable to concentrate on their schoolwork.

But you should continue to take them only under your doctor's supervision. Doses of amphetamines tend to grow larger, And Larger, AND LARGER.

Speed and Schoolchildren

Dear Dr. Schoenfeld:

I was taken aback by your seemingly approving comments on the use of drugs to facilitate studying in "problem" schoolchildren. Discussions of this type of program have appeared with some frequency in Science *and Hentoff's column in the* Village Voice. *It seems that this drugging of children may be disastrously close to good old cliché-ridden* 1984.

The positive alternative is to make the learning environment more responsive to the child rather than vice versa.

ANSWER: Amphetamines and amphetaminelike drugs such as methylphenidate hydrochloride (Ritalin) have been found useful in treating "hyperactive children." This is a relatively rare behavioral disorder. When administered under careful medical supervision, amphetamine-type drugs enable these children to focus their energies.

Undoubtably these same drugs are often misused to control normally active children bored by stultifying school routines which don't allow for individual differences.

Alcohol

A Dangerous Sedative

Dear Dr. Schoenfeld:

I have insomnia for weeks at a time, several times throughout the year. The rest of the time I sleep well.

I've tried mild sleeping pills, counting sheep, etc., but nothing short of drinking a six pack of beer every night gets me to sleep before 3 AM.

Any suggestions?

ANSWER: Since you have insomnia only at certain times during the year, you might try to examine your activities during these periods. Are you facing pressures from schoolwork or a job? Personal social problems perhaps?

Most people find that exercise followed by a warm bath gives relief from insomnia. Relying on drugs like alcohol or barbiturates for treating insomnia may lead to serious problems.

Alcohol and Impotence

Dear Dr. Hip Pocrates:

Recently you wrote several interesting paragraphs in answer to a man's inquiry about his impotence. You mentioned that liquor could be a contributing factor, I remember.

My husband is a very heavy drinker and to date has not found a sufficiently good reason to slow down or quit entirely, which would please me more. He seldom has an urge for lovemaking. When he does he is never able to consummate it, though at one time we had a very satisfactory relationship, physically.

What are the prospects for a man who loves his wife—if he refrains entirely from drinking? Is he likely again to enjoy going to bed with her and make her happy, too?

ANSWER: Impotence is among the many serious problems frequently associated with excessive use of alcohol. Fear of failure leads to further failures and the victim, paradoxically, may turn to alcohol for solace.

Alcoholism is best treated by individuals or groups experienced with this complex problem. The department of mental health of your local health department should be able to recommend help for your husband—if he's willing to accept it. Counseling or therapy might also be advisable for you. Many wives unwittingly contribute to their husband's alcoholism.

Narcotics

One of the reasons we are so far behind in the treatment of hard-core drug addiction is that it has always been viewed as a law-enforcement rather than a medical problem.

Sidney Malitz, M.D.
Chief of Psychiatric Research
New York Psychiatric Institute of
Columbia University
(*Hospital Tribune*, February 23, 1970)

The following letter, received in the fall of 1969, signaled the growing problem of narcotic addiction amongst U.S.

servicemen in Indochina. Not until 1971 did the Pentagon provide for drug amnesty and rehabilitation services.

Dear Dr. Schoenfeld:

I am presently in the U.S. Army and stationed in Vietnam. Although I had served one year here, I extended my duty time six months after a thirty-day leave in the United States. The reason I returned to Vietnam was because I found myself addicted to opium.

I thought that smoking opium couldn't cause addiction. I began smoking it about one year ago because of my close relationship to a Vietnamese. Since then, I have probably smoked one ounce every single day. During my leave, the small amount of opium I had with me soon disappeared. Twenty-four hours later, an ordeal of pain began which lasted until I returned to Vietnam two weeks later.

I've tried to give up opium by going "cold turkey" but this failed because of the pain. I've also tried the "ladder" bit by smoking a decreasing amount day by day. This didn't help either.

The symptoms are clear: everything from a running nose to an aching body. With four months' duty left you can imagine my concern. I even went as far as to ask advice of a team leader who is so straight that he almost got me busted. Turning myself into a military hospital is hopeless as it is an automatic bust by the MPs and the CID.

Is there any advice you could give me?

ANSWER: Opium is the parent compound of more potent narcotics such as heroin and morphine. Infrequent use of opium will not cause addiction. But regular use causes true addiction in a significant number of people.

Withdrawal from narcotics can either be done abruptly or gradually but many obstacles are still placed before addicts seeking treatment. Most hospitals refuse to treat narcotics addicts and those that do must often report these cases to police. Outpatient treatment of narcotics addicts in the United States is greatly restricted by federal law.

Military and V.A. hospitals now provide treatment for servicemen with drug-connected problems.

Narcotics withdrawal causes acute discomfort for several days. But the most difficult part is resisting further use. If your friends are all using the drug, you'll probably do the same.

$300 Daily Habit

Dear Dr. Schoenfeld:

Have you heard of the $300 a day heroin habit? I have but I can't understand it.

The price in my area for a balloon of smack is about $15, depending on quality. That fix lasts about six hours, so if you fixed every six hours, it would total about $50 a day.

This is all just approximate, but I am wondering if the $300 a day habit is truth or fiction.

ANSWER: Heroin is cut many times before it reaches the user. Even if street balloons contained a uniform amount (and they don't), the dose is gradually increased because of "tolerance."

A $300-a-day habit would be unlikely only because few addicts can afford to pay that much a day for their smack. But it's not unusual for an addict to steal $300 a day in marketable goods in order to support a sixty-dollar-a-day habit.

Shared syringes and needles often transmit serum hepatitis and this witless practice can communicate other diseases as well. An outbreak of malaria occurred in Bakersfield, California, in 1970, apparently the result of sharing "outfits" with servicemen returning from the Asian War.

Clinics and Privacy

Dear Dr. Schoenfeld:

I'm strung out on heroin. This doesn't seem to have any long-term advantages.

There are a good many places which offer help to addicts who wish to kick. But to the best of my knowledge, all of them ask the name of the patients and take photographs, etc. The confidential file always eventually becomes available to the law enforcers.

Rather than risk exposure I've been drifting along day to day. Is there a way to obtain assistance anonymously?

ANSWER: I've never heard of a drug clinic routinely photographing its patients but they will ask for his name and address.

If I were strung out on a drug and didn't want to be part of a computer bank, I might choose to use a different name and address for my clinic visits. Theoretically, a patient's files may not be released without his permission but theory and reality don't always coincide.

Milk Is Not for Shooting

Dick Fine, M.D., a former resident in internal medicine at the University of California Medical Center in San Francisco, reported the case of a 14-year-old girl advised by "friends" to shoot up milk to cure a bad heroin high. Folklore among junkies has it that intravenous milk is also good treatment for "smack" overdoses. But milk is for drinking, not shooting. Milk injected into the veins causes fluid to accumulate in the lungs and interferes with blood clotting.

The girl was brought to San Francisco's Mission Emergency Hospital near death. Pink froth was bubbling from her lungs. When an emergency tracheotomy (an opening in the windpipe) was performed, pink foam sprayed high in the air. The girl remained in the intensive care unit of the hospital for two weeks.

The best emergency street medicine for heroin O.D.s is pain, according to Skip Gay, M.D., of the Haight-Ashbury Drug Treatment Clinic. Injecting milk or salt water beneath the skin will inflict pain and help to arouse the patient. But should these substances enter the veins they may cause death. Heroin or other drug O.D.s require skilled medical attention.

Injecting anything into the veins can be extremely

hazardous. Bad reactions can result not only from the impure substances used but also from the needle if it has been used by another person. The virus of serum hepatitis is not killed by boiling water. The incubation period of the disease may be as long as six months. Thus many people may be infected by one needle before symptoms appear in any of them.

Hepatitis is a serious disease which affects the liver. The symptoms are fatigue, nausea, possibly vomiting, dark-colored urine, light-colored stools, itching and yellowing of the skin and whites of the eyes.

Heroin is the leading cause of death among 18- to 35-year-olds in New York City. Heroin overdoses killed more than 200 teenagers in that city alone in 1970. Typical of these deaths was that of a 17-year-old Barnard College freshman named Antoinette Dishman who sniffed heroin at a party and was found dead the next morning.

Heroin has been blamed for the tragic deaths of Jimi Hendrix and Janis Joplin. But Jimi and Janis knew about the dangers of heroin. Why then did they die? My guess is from a mixture of drugs. Large amounts of barbiturates were found in Jimi's blood and Janis was seldom seen without a bottle of booze. Alcohol, barbiturates or narcotics taken alone frequently lead to disastrous results. When combined they are even more dangerous.

Addiction in Unborn Babies

Dear Dr. Schoenfeld:

I am 5 months pregnant and I have sniffed small amounts of heroin a couple of times during the last month. The reason I am writing this to you is to find out whether or not this would have any effect on my pregnancy or the child's condition.

It is very important to me as I don't want to do anything to hurt my baby.

ANSWER: Heroin addiction is often found in babies born to female junkies. If it is undetected, the baby may die from withdrawal symptoms. Even if you haven't used enough smack to addict yourself or the fetus, each time you sniffed it, he was also narcotized. Moreover, heroin is frequently cut with quinine, a drug which could cause premature labor and delivery (but not abortions, despite popular belief). The chances are your baby remains healthy—keep it that way by stopping the use of all drugs during pregnancy.

Cocaine . . . Cocaine

Many people have asked about the effects of cocaine so I've sniffed out some information.

Cocaine stimulates the central nervous system, reduces hunger and, when applied directly to mucous membranes such as those lining the nose and mouth, produces anesthesia and constriction of blood vessels. The drug is derived from leaves of *Erythroxylon coca* and, for centuries, 90 percent of natives of Peru and Bolivia have chewed coca leaves for their stimulatory effect.

An article on Argentina appearing in a 1970 Braniff Airlines travel magazine recommends to adventurous tourists the local custom of chewing coca leaves after dining. Its author describes pleasurable tingling sensations of the mouth and tongue resulting from cocaine's anesthetic effects. Perhaps Braniff Airlines officials risk prison for using Madison Avenue techniques to promote pleasure through drugs.

Cocaine was first used in medicine by a young Viennese physician named Sigmund Freud. Freud experimented personally with cocaine for some time and apparently developed many of his theories of psychoanalysis aided by the drug. (Use of a drug to develop a drugless therapy is illustrated also by Synanon games, which are said to have evolved from an LSD experience.) Freud thought cocaine was a psychiatric wonder drug and prescribed it for virtually every mental illness.

He referred to cocaine as a "magical drug" and used it himself in "very small doses . . . regularly against depression and . . . indigestion." Freud found cocaine an aphrodisiac and described "the most gorgeous excitement" and "virility" it produced in him. He gave it to his fiancée, Martha Bernays, and wrote her, "You shall see who is the stronger, the gentle little girl who doesn't eat enough or a big, wild man who has cocaine in his body."

Many cases of cocaine poisoning among his patients, including one death, caused a public scandal. Freud stopped prescribing the drug for his patients but may have continued personal usage. His death was caused by a form of oral cancer. Whether or not chronic cocaine irritation caused the cancer we shall never know, but Freud is described as applying cocaine to the cancer toward the end of his life in order to relieve pain.

Cocaine is similar to amphetamines in many ways. Tolerance (the necessity to take more and more to achieve the same effect) develops easily and high doses can lead to a toxic paranoid psychosis. An overdose of cocaine may cause convulsions and death.

Intravenous use of cocaine seems rare today but sniffing the drug is once more in vogue. Cocaine sniffers may develop perforations of the nasal septum (the cartilage between the nostrils) due to contact tissue burns and constriction of local blood vessels resulting in tissue damage from lack of oxygen.

Cocaine is sometimes falsely classified as an addictive drug but withdrawal doesn't cause the abstinence symptoms seen in junkies. Once a habit has been established cocaine withdrawal may produce symptoms similar to those seen in withdrawal from amphetamines—depression, fatigue and listlessness.

Mixed Bag

Catnip

Dear Dr. Schoenfeld:

I've recently heard that smoking catnip is very similar to smoking marijuana. Could you tell me if there is any truth in this or is it a big put-on by the catnip industry to get you to buy their product?

ANSWER: A story in the *Wall Street Journal* reporting surging catnip sales around the country included information from a *Journal of the A.M.A.* article about catnip use by humans. A different kind of cat is using catnip these days and the *Wall Street Journal* notes the price of the tabby turn-on was only about 60¢ a lid. The *J.A.M.A.* subjects claimed catnip is nearly as potent as marijuana but the research division of the Telegraph Avenue Irregulars disputes this finding. My informants claim a catnip high is somewhere between dried banana peel linings and poor marijuana. Maybe there are grades of catnip like Calico Gold or Siamese Green. Is milk consumption also on the increase?

Stalking further information I telephoned Alexander "Sashe" Shulgin, Ph.D., the brilliant chemist who is best known to the public for his synthesis of STP (which was later illegally distributed in a dose form twice that "recommended").

"Sashe," I purred, "what can you tell me about catnip?"

He promised to send me some information and soon his letter arrived. Portions of it follow:

The plant is called catnip or catmint (*Nepeta cataria*). Steam distillation of the plant yields a volatile oil (about 0.3 percent) that is mostly acidic (inactive).

The volatiles seem to turn on members of the cat family only. McElvain screened his fractions using the lion as a test animal. There is some reputation of the use of catnip in humans, as a tea for nervous headache.

There is a report from Puerto Rico (1945) that catnip was detected as an adulterant in marijuana!

A number of other chemicals have been established as being present in catnip (as citral, geraniol, nerol, camphor, citronellol) but of some interest is the content of ascorbic acid.

. . . the active ingredient, nepetalactone.

The chemical . . . is completely unrelated to any known family of hallucinogens.

An extremely similar substance . . . is isolated from the Argentine ant, *Iridomyrmex humilis.*

. . . similar compounds are found in yet another insect, the stick insect, *Anisomorpha buprestoides.*

. . . if catnip smoking seems to lose its charm, one can always turn to cigarettes made of Argentine ants.

Maybe the person who coined the word *Roach* knew something that we don't.

Ground catnip closely resembles ground marijuana leaves. Nothing is known about possible harmful effects from short- or long-term use of the drug.

Supershuck

Dear Dr. Hip Pocrates:

I just ordered some "supergrass" as advertised in many of the underground papers and now I'm sort of worried. What is it that I've ordered?

Will it work? Is it dangerous having it mail-ordered to my house? Is it safe, health and head-wise? I'm hoping that it's good. At $1.50 a lid it would be nice . . .

ANSWER: You won't be busted and chances are you won't be stoned either. "Supergrass" is plain old catnip so give it to your cat. Maybe you'll get a contact high.

Oregano

Dear Dr. Schoenfeld:

Is there any documented information on the effects of oregano? I have smoked this spice and experienced a pleasant, mildly psychedelic tranquillity. Is this practice physically injurious?

Seasonably Stoned

ANSWER: Most people who are into spices believe the effects of smoking oregano are about like those of dried banana peel lining. That is, little or no effect. Some spices, like nutmeg or cinnamon, definitely have psychedelic effects when ingested but harm to the liver and kidneys may result.

Some historians believe that the spices sought by early explorers were valued for their mind-altering properties equally as much as their ability to preserve and flavor food.

More Spices

Dear Dr. Schoenfeld:

She said it made gaps in her mind—"the way grass does": smoking thyme with a pinch of oregano. Will such smoking produce permanent "gaps"?

ANSWER: Well it might affect her basil metabolism. . . .

PCP

Dear Dr. Schoenfeld:

Does PCP cause pinpoint brain lesions?

ANSWER: Not to my knowledge. PCP (Sernyl), an animal tranquilizer, is the usual component of capsules or tablets falsely sold as THC (tetrahydrocannabinol).

Mixed Drugs

Dear Dr. Schoenfeld:

I have a question to ask which has been worrying me.

Saturday night I made a 1000 microgram trip on white Owsley (LSD) and Sunday I made a trip on THC. This morning I woke up with my period. I'm always on time and I didn't expect it for ten more days. Could the acid be the reason for it? Do you think it has affected my system? This was only the 4th time I made acid.

ANSWER: Irregular periods are common during adolescence and at other times of emotional stress. Many female readers report drug usage has caused changes in their menstrual cycles. The cause is unknown. Perhaps it's the direct effect of the drug or the drugs may act indirectly by changing the female's emotional state. Almost always these are temporary changes.

Triad

Dear Dr. Schoenfeld:

What are the potential dangers of the new "3-way" tablets (mostly mescaline plus a little LSD and a wee bit of cocaine)?

One of my friends got stoned wild for 9 hours on this but spent the last 3 hours on the john. What's coming off?

ANSWER: Maybe your friend's intestinal lining. How can you be sure of the purity of these drugs? Or the dosage? Or even that they're the drugs you believe them to be?

Barbiturates

WARNING: The use of "reds" or barbiturates for highs (lows would be more descriptive) seems to be increasing again. Seconal (secobarbital) and Nembutal (pentobarbital) are two commonly prescribed medications often used in suicide attempts. Barbiturates are also physically addicting and kicking a barbiturate habit is more difficult and dangerous than kicking narcotics.

Mixing "reds" and alcohol can lead to a one-way trip because the two drugs potentiate each other, i.e., 1 + 1 = more than 2. In the case of barbiturates and alcohol the whole equals more than the sum of the parts.

Meprobamate

Dear Dr. Schoenfeld:

Please, is there anyplace or anything to stop a girl of 29 who has been taking meprobamate (Miltown, Equanil) tranquilizers for 8 years? She has been hospitalized. Can not be stopped. It didn't help. I am terrible afraid for her life. I do anything to get her out of it.

She had a psychiatrist for a time but it didn't help—she came home from his office and took them again—8 or 10 a day.

Her memory will be gone and finally death will come of it. Please Dr. could you advise something or some good place where she could not get to Miltown—even some private nice place. Best would be for her to go to a place where she can not get it. But not Synanon place.

Grieving Mother

ANSWER: Most people aren't aware that meprobamate (Equanil, Miltown) can be an addictive drug. That's one reason why it's only available through a physician's order.

Many communities with a large hip population have "Switchboards" which could refer your daughter to a treatment facility. Another source of information is the department of mental health of your local health department. You didn't say why Synanon was ruled out—it might be just the right kind of therapy for her.

Soapers

Dear Dr. Schoenfeld:

I would appreciate any information you have about a drug referred to as a "soaper": allegedly a simple, nonaddicting relaxant with a short-term reaction and no aftereffects.

ANSWER: "Soaper" comes from "Soper," one of the trade names for methaqualone, a drug now popular as a sedative and sleeping pill. Other trade names for methaqualone are Optimil, Parest, Quaalude and Somnafac.

Methaqualone quickly became a popular prescription drug because it was supposedly safe and nonaddictive. It quickly became a popular street drug because of the euphoria and sensual high produced. The *PharmChem Newsletter* states:

> After ingestion of 150 to 500 mg., the user first experiences a tingling sensation and his body becomes extremely relaxed (jellyfish). Inhibitions disappear. More candid, flowing communication creates a feeling of intimacy. The mood is conducive to sharing. Users have attributed aphrodisiacal properties to the drug, probably because of these physical and psychological effects. Extreme muscle relaxation makes it difficult to walk without stumbling. The individual may have trouble coordinating movement of his arms and legs. He also experiences difficulty talking; his speech is slow and slurred. Sleep usually follows in-

voluntarily, depending upon the individual and dosage. Undesirable side effects are usually absent when used under prescription.

Methaqualone is now known to be as dangerous and addictive as the barbiturates. Deaths have resulted from overdoses—most occurred when the drug was combined with alcohol. Convulsions are common when methaqualone addicts attempt to withdraw from the drug: for this reason withdrawal from methaqualone addiction should be conducted only in a hospital. How ironic that this "new barbiturate" has the same failings.

Methaqualone, like all the drugs we hear so much about, has beneficial properties if used properly. But misuse can be disastrous.

Laughing Gas

Dear Dr. Schoenfeld:

Recently, friends and I turned onto a drug popular with poets and literati generations ago, nitrous oxide. He found the experience to be among the most religious we have encountered with the strongest of the psychedelics. I could easily see how it could be called simply "laughing gas" but if one knows where to go, it can take you to the void, the threshold of death, "IT," "Ohm" or whatever it all means to you.

Anyway, we took in alternate tokes of N_2O and air, passing the tank around the room or sometimes taking two or three hits consecutively until either we were too far beyond to handle the mechanical valve, or until it was felt that we might not be getting enough oxygen to the brain anymore.

Thus my question is, what are the potential dangers in-

volved in the use of nitrous oxide this way? Would a person become anesthetized before damage would occur?

Om Shanti

ANSWER: Nitrous oxide was a popular turn-on for medical students at least as early as 1808. Later in the nineteenth century, carnival sideshows offered "laughing gas" at 5¢ a whiff. Today N_2O is one of the most widely used anesthetics and it's a curious fact that almost every person who has had a general anesthetic, i.e., "put to sleep," has gone on a far-out psychedelic trip.

The chief danger in the use of nitrous oxide for highs is death by asphyxiation. This could occur if a person strapped an anesthesia mask around his head, attached it to the tank, and turned the tank and himself on. Death is caused not from the effects of the gas but from lack of oxygen while the person is unconscious.

Another common danger, and one greatly feared by anesthetists, could be caused by eating just before using the gas. Nitrous oxide causes a significant number of people to be nauseated, and vomiting while under the effects of the gas could cause food to be aspirated into the lungs. Taking the gas directly from the tank might cause painful freezing of the lips or possibly the larynx.

Other dangers are theoretically possible but uncommon. Nothing is known about possible harm from chronic use of nitrous oxide.

No Laughing Matter: Cyclopropane

Word is some folks use the anesthetic cyclopropane (Trimethylene) for their highs. I hope this message reaches you in time.

Cyclopropane is far more dangerous than laughing gas. Arrhythmias of the heart and respiratory failure are not uncommon effects. In other words, the heart may stop beating or beat so quickly and weakly that blood is not circulated through the body. The brain centers which control breathing may be so heavily anesthetized that breathing stops. These emergencies can be dealt with in an operating room by trained anesthetists and surgeons. If they happen elsewhere your best hope is a groovy reincarnation.

Nausea and vomiting often follow use of cyclopropane. If a person is zonked out and vomits, he is likely to aspirate the partially digested food into his lungs, another way to go out in a hurry. Cyclopropane is also explosive and several operating room explosions and fires have resulted from its use. If you're still tempted to use cyclopropane for kicks after reading this, it's plain you're seeking suicide, not nirvana.

A Tale of Karma

A California State Narcotics agent was beaten senseless by San Francisco police and sent to the county hospital. The 26-year-old, bearded, long-haired agent was caught by accident in a dope raid. When he reached inside his coat for identification, the police thought he was going for a gun so they grabbed and frisked him. He did have a gun. Splat! When the police stopped working him over, he had two deep scalp lacerations, red welts all over his back and was semiconscious. When he was finally able to identify himself, he was sent to a ward of San Francisco General Hospital which treats public employees.

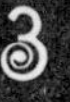

Sex, Drugs and Treason

. . . a four-year course in sex, drugs and treason.

Max Rafferty, Ph.D., commenting on the University of California at Berkeley during his term as California's Superintendent of Public Instruction. Eugene Schoenfeld was a staff physician for Berkeley's Student Health Service from 1966 to 1970.

Moses Hall

The first of the casualties came before any confrontation. A girl with a lacerated toe.

"How did it happen?" I asked.

"Oh, I was jumping from a barricade and must of caught my foot on a nail." She was short and plump* and good-humored.

"Were you barefooted?"

"No, I was wearing sandals," she sighed.

The wound was beneath and on the side of the fourth toe. After the nurse cleaned her foot, I anesthetized and sutured the toe. Just a few nylon sutures required, but a difficult area in which to work. The girl had received a tetanus toxoid booster within the past year so didn't need another. One less jabbing.

We had been alerted to the possibility of many injuries. Several of the nurses worked a double shift that night. Three or four staff physicians were on call at home, ready to come to the hospital if needed. We waited.

Another student with an injured toe, this time a tall slender fellow with camera slung over his shoulder. He'd been taking photographs for the *Daily Californian.*

"How did it happen?" I asked.

"I jumped from a barricade." One of his toes was dislocated, jutting out at a strange angle. I injected an anesthetic, reduced the dislocation, and ordered X rays in the morning.

* I ran into this girl later at a People's Park demonstration. She told me that she'd gone on a diet after reading my "plump" remark.

"That looks better," he said. The nurse taped the toe to an adjacent one and he hobbled out of the hospital.

We waited. The hospital administrator returned from the campus police station and sat down at the second floor nurses' station. He looked worried.

"Man oh Man," he said, "they are really mad."

The second sit-in in a week. Sproul Hall a few days ago and now Moses. Some of the police were thumping their nightsticks against tables and walls.

I went upstairs to the doctors' quarters and tried to sleep. Maybe I did for an hour or so. At 6 A.M. the telephone rang.

"Doctor, there are four or five state highway patrolmen in the dispensary. One has blood coming from his mouth." I dressed and went downstairs.

Three uniformed policemen were in the emergency room, one lying on the operating table. His mouth was covered with blood.

"How did it happen?" I asked.

"Hit by a brick," he replied.

One of his front teeth was chipped. The blood came from a small laceration inside his upper lip.

"Do you have a dentist?"

"Yes."

"Better see him tomorrow." The nurse gave him a tetanus booster.

A student entered the emergency room, holding a blood-soaked handkerchief to his forehead. He glared momentarily at the cop lying a few feet away.

I removed the handkerchief from his forehead and saw a jagged laceration about an inch and a half in length.

"What happened?"

"I guess I didn't move fast enough or something. I was just on the sidelines watching and was hit with a billy club." I ordered skull X rays.

More police entered the dispensary. A senior staff physician joined me. She looked at the scene (which now resembled a disaster area) and shook her gray head sadly.

One of the uniformed men lay on a table too narrow for his girth. He was an old man with a huge belly and obviously had been called out of retirement.

"What happened to you?"

"Hit in the ribs with a brick." The X rays showed no fracture but I knew this to be a painful injury from my own memories of a kick in the ribs long ago. I gave him a codeine preparation for pain.

Most of the injuries were contusions and abrasions. Bruises and scrapes. One young highway patrolman had a laceration of his shin. Another brick.

As I sutured the wound he said, "Man, will I be glad to go home. My wife and kids haven't seen me in four days."

"Yeah," another patrolman cracked, "we spend so much time at this university they should give us degrees."

The skull films of the injured student were ready now. He joined the gray-haired doctor and me as we looked for fracture lines.

"Gee, is that me?" he asked, cheerful once more.

We saw no fracture. When I finished suturing his forehead the day staff was arriving at the hospital. I changed clothes, left the hospital and walked across the campus to Moses Hall. Some of my friends had been inside the building and were now in jail.

Workmen were removing the last of the barricades. A professor stood beside his bicycle arguing with a student. Office girls were outside the building picking up papers strewn from file cabinets. The work of students, said the police. The work of the police, said the students.

Overhead a news helicopter circled and recircled, filming the scene for television's most popular show.

The Battle for People's Park

Dan Siegal, president-elect of Cal's student body, said he never finished his talk to the thousands gathered to rally behind the Berkeley People's Park. When he suggested they take the park, avoiding bloodshed and arrest, the crowd immediately left Sproul Plaza. Chanting "We want the park," and whooping like Indians, they spilled out onto Telegraph Avenue and walked to the Haste Street intersection where a line of helmeted, brown-uniformed police waited behind barricades.

For a few minutes demonstrators and police eyed each other warily. The chanting continued and a few students taunted the police. Suddenly a fire hydrant on the northwest corner was opened sending a graceful arc of water cattycorner across the intersection. Some street people soon changed the direction of the arc, drenching the police and causing the only laughter heard that day.

Rocks and bottles appeared next, flipping end over end, crashing down on both police and demonstrators. I heard a noise to my right and turned in time to see a charging squad of burly men in powder-blue jump suits. "Blue Meanies," specially chosen for their size, strength and utter dedication to the rule of club and gun. They raced to the fire hydrant, scattering students who slipped and fell in the wet intersection. Now the first tear gas canisters were thrown, driving most of the demonstrators up Telegraph and into the side streets. Another group retreated toward Dwight Way.

Confrontations with tear gas are short-lived if you don't have a mask. I held my breath as long as I could and turned up Channing Way. Just ahead of me an Oriental girl and her crew-cut blond male friend were gasping and choking—a tear gas canister had exploded at their feet. They were taken to a nearby residence hall.

I continued up Channing Way and literally ran into Sergio Scherr hurrying to the Avenue to take photos for father Max's *Barb*.

"Are you all right, man?" he asked. My eyes were bright red and tears streamed down my cheeks but I hadn't been badly gassed. Sergio continued on to the Avenue while I looked for some cool tap water. My cheeks were beginning to sting. A secretary unlocked the door to a university office building and three of us headed for a sink. We washed our eyes and faces with soothing cool water, taking care not to rub in the clinging gas.

Outside the building the streets were still fairly quiet. Students strolled slowly up and down Channing Way looking through parking lots at the People's Park on Haste Street. Most of the demonstrators returned to Telegraph but were soon driven up the street to the busy Durant intersection. No one had bothered to block traffic and scores of frightened drivers were temporarily trapped in their cars. Some of the students argued about blocking off the street. One had the ingenious idea of directing autos the wrong way, down Telegraph and into the police lines.

"Let these drivers find out about tear gas," he said. But the first car in the right lane was a Cadillac driven by a terrified Little Old Lady and she wouldn't go any direction but forward. Smart move. A huge dump truck roared across the intersection barely missing several demonstrators. Its cursing driver ducked a small volley of wadded paper and fruit.

A few rocks and bottles were hurled from Durant toward the police on Channing Way.

"We ought to be throwing bullets, not bottles," someone said.

"Cool it, man," his friend replied.

The police charged to the Durant intersection. Fleeing demonstrators or the police knocked down an elderly white-haired lady in front of Larry Blake's Restaurant. Several students huddled about her long slender form stretched full length on the sidewalk. I walked across Telegraph intending to help her but was met by an eerie sight, an armed figure peering through his gas mask and waving a club.

"Get out of here," he shouted through the mask.

"I'm a doctor and I want to help that woman."

He ran toward me club extended and I split. The old woman was helped to her feet and limped to the lines of the demonstrators. Hanging from her neck was a handwritten sign saying, "I *love* the People's Park." I flashed on the last time I had been in the park—children playing on the swings, David Scherr (another of Max's sons) working with pick and shovel planting a tree, the distribution of free food.

Dense clouds of tear gas now billowed up from the Telegraph-Dwight area. An unmarked police car was overturned and burned and the police drove the crowds south on Telegraph. My laboratory assistant was on Ward and Telegraph when she attempted to escape the gas by running into a small building on a lot owned by Cunha Pontiac. One of the Cunha Pontiac employees drove her out shouting, "Get out, get out, you deserve everything you're getting." I suppose she said the same when their showrooms were later destroyed.

Jeeps with police literally riding shotgun weaved up and down Telegraph apparently trying to run down students. Sawed-off shotguns carrying heavy lead slugs (not the birdshot initially reported by police) were used to gun down anyone in sight. A 24-year-old carpenter on the roof of the Telegraph Repertory Theater was hit in the face by a shotgun blast. He will be blind for life.

Another shotgun blast ripped through the abdomen of a 25-year-old man who was taken in critical condition to Herrick Hospital's intensive care unit. He lost his spleen, a large portion of his intestines and his left kidney. Later he died. Most of the people wounded by shotguns were released after treatment at Herrick Hospital. Ten were admitted, four in serious condition.

Cal's Student Health Service admitted ten students with gunshot wounds. Four had been shot with large bore slugs; two had through-and-through wounds of the extremities; one was hit in the shoulder and one in the abdomen.

One of the Cal students who was shotgunned worked in the hospital record room and often brought me patients' charts. He lost several fingers of his left hand.

A scene observed by Carolyn Winter during one of the People's Park skirmishes seemed to sum up the situation in Berkeley during those weeks. Standing in the middle of the Telegraph and Durant intersection was a heavily armed policeman clad in flak jacket and gas mask. From the corner of his eye he saw a sudden movement. Whirling around he heaved a tear gas grenade—at a small brown bird.

I left Telegraph Avenue when the police began their shooting. At the same moment James Rector lay mortally wounded on a rooftop, I was making love.

Old Glory—New Art

The audience stared incredulously at Old Glory. Their eyes moved down the little wooden staff and remained fixed on its base, a candle in the shape of an erect penis. The candle was red, white and blue and larger than life. Silver stars covered blue scrotum.

The flag-topped candle remained on the podium during my talk at a VD Teach-In held at the University of California's San Francisco Medical Center. Its creator, Jon Stedman, had been busted a few days earlier on Berkeley's Telegraph Avenue. He was charged with displaying obscene material, disgracing the flag and vending without a license. Bail was set at $800.

"As long as this part of the human body is considered obscene, we won't be able to eradicate venereal diseases," I told the assembled public health workers.

A week earlier, I had stopped at a tiny shop just across the street from Berkeley's People's Park to rap for a few minutes with Byron The Jeweler.

While looking at the rings my eyes caught the Stars and Stripes in the display case. It was a Jon Stedman objet d'art.

"Where did you get it?" I asked with patriotic zeal. Byron pointed across the street to a fellow near the entrance of a parking lot once part of People's Park.

I crossed Dwight Way and walked to the entrance of the parking lot where the candlemaker was talking to a group of pickets. Inside his van were several colored phallic candles but all his red, white and blue models had been snatched up by flag-waving Berkeleyans.

"I have more at home," Stedman told me. "I'll leave one for you at Byron's later today."

When I told Byron another show of the flag could be expected, he offered me his own candle. Returning to my bus I heard the usual sounds of Telegraph Avenue.

"Acid, grass, mescaline?"

The night before the VD Teach-In I read that Jon Stedman had been arrested. Whether or not he was vending without a license I can't say. But displaying obscene material? Only if our bodies are obscene. Disgracing the flag? Only if our bodies are disgraceful.

The Indochina War disgraced the flag. By comparison, Stedman's candle honors the flag. Long may it wave.

Alcatraz

Alcatraz. Its name evokes images from dozens of Grade B prison films. As a child I saw films of smoke pouring from the island during the 1946 prison riot, which ended only with the landing and use of the United States Marines. Many times I sailed past the island, never allowed closer than the 200-yard clearance required by the Coast Guard. That's why things didn't seem quite real as I sat outside a solitary confinement cell on Alcatraz. The cell contained medical supplies for the American Indians who occupied the island.

Indian children played at the other end of the cellblock, swinging from a rope tied to bars on the second tier of cells. (The twelve-year-old daughter of Indian leader Richard Oakes* fell to her death from one of these tiers.) Many of the cells were in use again, blankets on the bars giving privacy never enjoyed by former inmates.

"You want to see where Al Capone stayed?"

The Indians quickly learned Alcatraz lore. I had seen Capone's home in Miami Beach where he spent his last years and, yes, wanted to see the cell. The young red man pointed to the third tier of the main row, a cell exactly like the others. Scarface Al Capone was said to have bought preferential treatment during his years on the Rock. But no material goods, nothing bought with money could have much relieved the conditions of men imprisoned on the island. The Indians placed a carved American Eagle over the main entrance to the cell block and beneath the eagle a sign, "Land of the Free." But nowhere on the island can one really feel free. Not yet. Maybe not ever.

One of the few Anglos on the island, a young filmmaker, told a new Indian friend of his desire to take peyote while on Alcatraz. The answer was quick. "You crazy, man? Do you know what kind of spirits are here?" What kind of spirits were left by men whose cages were ten feet long by six feet wide? I entered one of the solitary confinement cells and pulled the heavy steel door closed. Blackness. When the prison functioned, some light could enter the cell through holes punched in the back wall, if the guards allowed it.

The "lucky" prisoners worked in one of the two Kafka-

* Oakes was shot to death in a "trespassing" incident in 1972.

like factories or the laundry or kitchen. But everywhere there were watchtowers and sagging catwalks. Rusting remnants of barbed wire surround the western side of the island near the cold bay waters. Only a few years had passed since the prisoners were transferred to other penitentiaries, yet most of the structures were nearly destroyed by the salt air, wind and seas.

I had never been within a prison before. Once I visited the concentration camp at Dachau. No gas ovens were on Alcatraz but it was the same experience.

The exercise yard was the main eating area for the Indians. Rust marks run down the high walls. A pup tent was set up on the small patch of scrub brush left uncovered by concrete. Sitting on the great cement steps, some of the Indians spoke of painting murals on the walls of the exercise yard. Plans were also made for giant tepees.

"Bad as Alcatraz is, it's better than many of the reservations." You heard this over and over from the Indians. They invoked an 1868 treaty between the Sioux and the U.S. Government that stipulates unused federal land reverts to the Indians.

The federal government declared Alcatraz surplus property and offered the island to San Francisco. Texas oilman H. L. Hunt proposed a futuristic monument and commercial exploitation. His plans were accepted by the S.F. Board of Supervisors on the recommendation of Mayor Joseph Alioto. But Alvin Duskin, a civic-minded dress manufacturer, ran a full page newspaper advertisement which expressed the feelings of most people in the San Francisco Bay Area. Why rush ahead with these plans so obviously unworthy of San Francisco and Alcatraz? The Board of Supervisors reversed its vote after a deluge of mail and telephone calls.

History has given us few pleasant surprises these last few years. The Indian occupation of Alcatraz was an exception. Public sentiment in S.F. overwhelmingly favored giving Alcatraz to the Indians. An Indian cultural and exhibition center could allow the display and perhaps sale of Indian art and craftwork. Millions of visitors to San Francisco would want to visit such a center and also see the old cellblock. They would learn at firsthand of the need for prison reform or elimination. No better use of Alcatraz Island has been or is likely to be proposed.

The last of the Indians were removed by federal marshals in June 1971.

Altamont or How to Produce a ~~Rock Concert~~ Disaster

1. Promise a free concert by a popular rock group which rarely appears in this country. Announce the site only four days in advance.
2. Change the location 20 hours before the concert.
3. The new concert site should be as close as possible to a giant freeway.
4. Make sure the grounds are barren, treeless, desolate.
5. Don't warn neighboring landowners that hundreds of thousands of people are expected. Be unaware of their out-front hostility toward long hair and rock music.
6. Provide 1/60 the required toilet facilities to insure that people will use nearby fields, the sides of cars, etc.
7. The stage should be located in an area likely to be completely surrounded by people and their vehicles.
8. Build the stage low enough to be easily hurdled. Don't secure a clear area between stage and audience.
9. Provide an unreliable barely audible low fidelity sound system.
10. Ask the Hell's Angels to act as "security" guards.

The Rolling Stones' free concert was touted as a Woodstock West. Another gathering of the New Culture. Further proof that hundreds of thousands of people could gather together, smoke dope and groove on music peacefully if only they weren't hassled by the Establishment.

I couldn't go to the Woodstock festival. That same weekend I was chairman of a panel on LSD and chromosomes at a University of California LSD symposium. So I missed Woodstock and got Altamont instead.

Prelude to a Bummer

We left Berkeley at two in the morning, Edward the Bear and Goldie Lox, retired groupie Diane, and myself. Traffic the next day was certain to be a drag so we decided to drive out at night and sleep in my bus.

The Altamont Speedway is about fifty miles from Berkeley. On the way you pass the Santa Rita prison farm and Livermore, home of fine wineries and a nuclear weapons factory. The road to Altamont was poorly marked and we passed the speedway area on our first try. Looking back we saw some cars parked on the freeway shoulder and two guys peeing against the hillside. Beyond them and over the hill were banks of lights, bonfires and buses. I turned the bus around, headed for the lights and soon found myself on Interstate 580 bound for Los Angeles. The speedway lights were to our right now. We pulled off the highway, drove through a field and up a hill followed by a funky 1938 Chevy sedan and several other buses. Reaching the crest we found ourselves on the rim of an irregular natural amphitheater.

Someone described the setting that night as resembling the circus scene from *"8½"* or the miracle scene from *La Dolce Vita.* Anyway, it was a Fellini trip. Eerie but groovy. Hundreds of occupied sleeping bags. Sounds of hammers. A derrick hoisted giant speakers to scaffolds on both sides of the stage.

We had just walked down the hill when I saw some people pointing to my right. I turned to see Mick Jagger approaching, followed by some cameramen. He stopped a few feet from us and watched the derricks.

A girl left her sleeping bag and ran to Mick. "I have a present for you," she said, smiling.

We thought for a moment *she* was the present, just as Diane had been once in an L.A. hotel. Diane and a girlfriend had dressed as maids and taken an elevator to the Stones' penthouse suite. Tales of poppers and endless fucking . . .

But this girl ran back to her sleeping bag and returned with a yellow knit scarf, placing it around Jagger's neck. December nights near Livermore are damned cold. I think he must have appreciated the warmth of the scarf as much as the girl's thoughtfulness. He thanked her and moved on. The rest of us enjoyed the whole scene. We couldn't know moments like that would be rare.

Behind the stage we ran into a merry crew from underground rock station KSAN-FM. They were trying to keep warm in Step Ponic's bus, one of the ubiquitous VWs.

Inside the KSAN Remote Unit–Ponic family bus was Gaby Ponic sipping some white wine, "Scoop" Nisker gathering items for radio's best news show, and sound man Paul Boucher, who bravely put a microphone in our midst. Paul asked about medical provisions for the concert. I hadn't found the medical tent yet but knew there was a crew of volunteer physicians and medics. Several psychiatry residents from the University of California Medical Center were also on the grounds by then, including my brother, Frank.

Edward the Bear was asked to give a few general impressions of Altamont.

"Sex—dope—sex—dope—sex—dope—sex—dope . . ."

The KSAN bus was parked in some kind of audio "hole" preventing them from hearing their station and Dusty Street's program. We lent them a portable which could pick up the station when placed on the bus roof. Cheery sounds then came from inside and outside the bus. They were in high spirits. Very high spirits.

I walked up the road and to the right where I found the medical tent set against the outer wall of the speedway stadium. Propane heaters took some of the chill from the air. Medical volunteers were in sleeping bags but awake and cheerful. We talked for a while. I thought that even with hundreds of thousands of people expected there wouldn't be many medical problems given a population so young and healthy and a concert scheduled for only five hours. I was wrong, of course. Michel Helms, one of the medical volunteers, told me a bad trip tent had been set up outside by the psychiatry residents. I couldn't find the trip tent in the darkness so returned to the stage area.

Bear and I walked about the grounds for a while trying to decide on the best spot for our bus. At the time there was still room behind the stage but the stage was in a gully we knew would soon be jammed with people. Finally we decided to stay on the hill. Thanks to karma and a guy peeing by the side of the highway, we had found the most peaceful spot at Altamont.

A few days earlier, Mimi Farina had asked why conversations inevitably turned to the excretory processes.

"Well," psychiatrist Bill Alexander observed, "conversational topics may run dry, but there's always shit to talk about." Talmudic-Freudian wisdom.

Saturday Morning

I awoke to pleasant tinkling noises (speaking of tinkling) coming from the stage. A Hare Krishna group, this generation's Salvation Army band.

From the front window I could see a huge hot-air balloon and the grounds rapidly filling with people. Except for the November 1969 Moratorium march in Washington, I had never seen a crowd so large—and more were coming.

Bear and Goldie placed a red blanket on the ground in front of the bus. To their left at the edge of the crowd I saw long lines waiting in front of portable toilets. Maybe that's one reason why things turned out as they did at Altamont. Pack 300,000 people together when they can't relieve themselves easily and you've got one uptight mean group.

There are no instruments to measure the kind of vibrations I picked up on leaving the bus. I felt them immediately and they were all bad. Why? I have some ideas.

Outdoor festivals should be held at a pleasant site, right? This one was outside a race-car track in barren fields next to a monster freeway. Most of the day was cold and gray with warmth provided neither from the skies nor the people.

Whenever a good thing began, it seemed to fizzle out. Multicolored coffee can lids were tossed like Frisbees for a while. But it didn't last. Nor did the sun which warmed us briefly in the afternoon, then faded.

The Concert

Santana led off the concert at noon, an hour ahead of schedule. The sound quality was poor but then the audio of even a medium-cost hi-fi system is superior to any outdoor concert I've ever attended. For most it's enough to see the groups and be together.

"Besides," Bear said sardonically, "we're helping to make history."

Our blanket was surrounded by people prepared for a good time. Wine, sandwiches and joints were freely shared. A Chicano tossed dozens of tangerines from a crate to the cheers of the crowd. Our part of the hillside, at least, tried to be happy and friendly early in the afternoon, but we never really made it.

Fights around the stage were first visible to us while the Airplane was playing. An English voice (Sam Cutler) kept asking people to clear the stage. Later he announced that Marty Balin had been decked by one of the Angels. From that time on fear grew and spread in the crowd. No one onstage except for some of the groups helped to dispel those feelings.

My "laboratory assistant," Jeanne, was sitting beneath a scaffold near the stage. She said the first hassle didn't involve Hell's Angels. A 300-pound middle-aged man stripped and walked in front of the stage. Several girls were dancing to the music, one of them a pretty blond Cal student named Renee, a fantastic dancer often seen in Berkeley's Sproul Plaza or Provo Park.

The 300-pound nude man walked up to Renee and kicked her in the chest. She sat down. Things got heavier from that time on.

Many people had taken impure LSD, or mixed reds with alcohol or speed. All potential bummers anyway but the chances of a bad trip are infinitely increased in a huge unhappy fear-ridden crowd.

Jeanne saw people who seemed to enjoy running through, over, and on wall-to-wall people. They freaked out completely on reaching the stage.

The Hell's Angels had been asked to act as a kind of security guard. Later they said they were promised $500 in beer just to sit on the stage. I believe they would have been content to drink beer and groove on the music if the mood around them had been peaceful. But it wasn't. And the Angels can just as easily groove on violence. Their method of treating drug freakouts was to club and gouge with cuesticks.

Maybe the Stones and their road manager, Sam Cutler, didn't really know the Angels' trip. Many people abroad have the idea they are a kind of jolly Robin Hood-like band.

Bad Trips

The bad trips began to "peak" at noon. So many freakouts occurred around the stage, a place was cleared on the ground behind the KSAN bus. Conditions were incredibly poor there for treating disturbed patients but there was no place else to go. Reaching the main hospital tent took 30 minutes when possible at all. A huge generator roared 20 feet away from the trip clearing and people wandered through freely.

Nearby, the driver of one of four Red Cross mobile units tried to move his vehicle out of the area. He'd realized vehicles would be useless trapped near the stage.

One physician told me it took 30 minutes just to have *calls* for medical attention relayed to the stage.

A medic led a short pudgy guy to the area. He was trembling and kept saying, "Give me some Thorazine. Give me some Thorazine. I want to come down." We sat him against a car bumper and started talking him down. Almost any tranquilizer will help treat a bad LSD trip but it's best not to use them, if possible. Some drugs sold as LSD turn out to be either impure or chemicals which mix badly with tranquilizers.

I left the stage area and skirted the edge of the audience in order to reach the medical tent. Half the tent was occupied by people on bad trips, most of them lying quietly on cots or the ground. Others yelled and cried.

Dr. Dick Fine of the Medical Committee for Human Rights was in charge of the medical facility. We had just begun to talk when a Red Cross ambulance pulled up. Attendants carried a patient into the tent. His right eye was swollen shut. Blood trickled from a laceration over the eye. The rest of his face was swollen and bruised. Dr. Fine began asking him questions to determine his mental status.

"What day is this?"

"Thursday."

"What month is it?"

"November."

Wrong answers mumbled through split lips.

The beatings took place around the stage but waves of terror and anger seemed to ripple through the massive audience.

Late in the afternoon I ran across Bill Alexander, K.O. Hallinan, Mimi Farina and Milan Melvin. Sure they'd felt the vibes. They picked up their blanket and split before the Stones began.

Near the trip tent I saw the Hog Farm's Hugh Romney (Wavy Gravy). We had starved together at the Liferaft Earth Hunger Show before I was done in by a waffle.

"It's not Woodstock," said Wavy Gravy.

Hearing the sounds of motorcycles, I looked up and saw

several Angels getting ready to go to the stage by moving their bikes through 300,000 people. Sonny Barger described the ride during a long telephone monologue on KSAN the following night. The Angels drove their bikes in low gear, almost walking them down. Most people managed to move out of the way but one girl muttered something like "fucking Angels." As Barger told it, one of the Angels said to his woman, "You gonna let her talk to us like that?" She left the motorcycle, belted the offending female and mounted the bike again. They passed through the audience and parked their bikes in front of and to the side of the stage.

Now it was dusk. Outside the trip tent, a tall, well-dressed 18- or 19-year-old black fellow talked with two Langley Porter psychiatry residents.

"I want to go back to Berkeley," he said. "Someone put drugs in my food. I'm scared."

I looked into the faces of people as I walked back to my bus. A lot of us were scared.

I reached the bus just as the Rolling Stones were announced.

Mick Jagger tried but couldn't stop the fighting. I wasn't taking notes and can't remember how many times Jagger stopped the performance to plead for peace or ask for a doctor. Without binoculars we could barely distinguish individual figures. Only Jagger was easily visible, dancing in his crimson costume beneath the spotlights.

Several times we saw what appeared to be a group of figures dressed in black charge from the stage into the crowd. Sonny Barger said several of the Angels' motorcycles were jostled or pushed over by the crowd surging around the stage. Enraged Angels "got" anyone suspected of damaging the bikes. An Angel's bike, Barger explained, means more to him than anything else on earth. During one of the stage brawls, an 18-year-old black youth was killed, gun in hand, stabbed five times in the back and once in the neck. The Angels said he had threatened Mick Jagger.

Finally, the concert ended. Most cars were parked miles from the speedway. We turned around, drove downhill and were on the freeway in a few minutes. The concert ended at 8 P.M. By 9:30 I was home.

How to sum up the whole experience?

When you feel a sense of relief on arriving home safely from a concert, when you call friends and relatives to make sure they're safe as well, when soaking in a hot bath doesn't help your head as it usually will—you know you've been through a giant bummer. This one was called Altamont.

The Powder Hill Rock Festival (A Mother's Report)

Dearest ——,

Daddy came up this weekend; I hadn't expected him this week but he said that it was so hot at home that he just had to get away from the heat.

What a mess is going on in Middlefield. Powder Hill Ski people leased their place to the people who run the Rock and Roll Festivals. Suddenly, Middlefield was besieged with so many awful characters that the residents sought an injunction which was granted by the court. The Festival cannot be held; however, the people are still here, some of the most horrible characters according to the newspaper pictures and the wide coverage on television. In last night's Press there are many pictures of them going into the pond nude; the papers and TV cannot show the pictures of them in the nude; so they do the next best thing; show the pictures of them from the rear; one was a girl holding a baby walking into the water.

They won't leave Middlefield. The State Police are stationed at the boundaries; no car permitted, but they are walking in and going in over the mountain, walking. The conservative estimate is 25,000, but they say that there are more and more going in. Last night's commentator reported that hepatitis has broken out and skin rashes so the pool has been closed; one girl gave birth to a baby yesterday. Drug pushers are working in the open; over 200 of the people there already have been admitted to the hospital; and the Middlesex always is overcrowded as it is.

Since you are such a liberal, I wish you would tell us what these longhaired, bearded, barefoot characters are trying to prove. Most of them are filthy; their hair, beards, feet and clothes are filthy. Does that prove anything? And does it prove anything to vandalize, to overrun decent communities, go on drug binges, and—oh yes—open sex. And they're all screaming about justice. Did Daddy and I and parents like us do anything worse than to overindulge our children; to deny ourselves things we wanted to give you (and I say this plurally—for us and parents like us), a wonderful education, allowances so that you would have enough to eat and be independent; yes, be independent? I hope and pray, fervently, that you don't go along with—and don't condone—this hooliganism that is going on. It's disgusting, it's discouraging, and it's just terribly upsetting. Middlefield is a beautiful New England village, a quiet bucolic village; just what is it going to look like when all those filthy pigs get out of there? Lyman's orchards are suffering, too; people can't get over there to buy peaches, etc. I just hope that they won't raid the orchards; it isn't unlikely.

Well, enough of that. It's showery and cloudy today which is too bad. We have had such beautiful weather all summer; I'd like it to be nice for Daddy and for the ———s. However, the prediction is for a beautiful day tomorrow. I'll still go in for my swim in the rain. Hate to miss a day; I say my daily swim is therapeutic for me. Always said that, didn't I? Everyone loves your picture.

Mrs. ——— said that you are very thin. Please eat well and do eat lots of nourishing food. How about lots of fattening food?

Much love from Daddy and me.

The Movement Meets the Media

What was the Alternative Media Conference? Beats hell out of me. I doubt if any one person yet knows or will ever know. Maybe Mike Rossman or someone can assemble the tapes, writings, cartoons and photographs which resulted in some kind of coherent impression. Maybe. For me it was a five-day kaleidoscope of 2000 media and movement freaks and Vermont which began, appropriately enough, with a benefit for *The Realist*'s fictitious Tenth Anniversary issue.

Esalen had massaged Paul Krassner's mind and bod and he talked for three hours at San Francisco's New Committee Theater about Big Sur and the Chicago Conspiracy trial.

Much of Krassner's talk centered around the split between him and Abbie Hoffman and Jerry Rubin. The ostensible reason was Paul's dropping LSD just before he testified at the Conspiracy trial. But obviously that wasn't all of it. The trial was a farce anyway. The real reason was the polarization tearing at all of us. That's what much of the Alternative Media Conference was about—I think.

After Paul's talk I was introduced to Dick Rosenblatt who told of something called the Alternative Media Conference to be held at Goddard College in Vermont. Chartered plane leaving in two days. Did I want to go? Why not. Rosenblatt said he'd leave my name at the gate.

Up early Tuesday morning I write a column in near-record time, drop off column newspaper-bound, drop by dark-haired beauty's house for awkward tea, she crying as I leave and my tears saved for later while I watched my ex-laboratory assistant/old lady absorbed in a recipe book. "Why?" she asked in wonder later at the heliport. "Love for you welling from my eyes," I told her. And then I was off to the San Francisco airport and she to Oregon.

Mike Korman, formerly with Pacifica's KPFA, and dress manufacturer–conservationist Alvin Duskin rode next to me in the helicopter for the ten-minute ride over the magnificent bay. We exchanged our zilch knowledge about the Media Conference but figured the plane ride would be literally out of sight. Tooling up to the United Airlines gate, we gave our names and were waved through.

The plane was nearly full by the time we entered. Full of the freakiest passengers ever assembled in one aircraft. Bob McClay and Mary Turner from KSAN-FM, Bob Prescott and Joshua from KMPX-FM, Paul Krassner, Sam Silver from *Good Times*, Ronnie Davis of the S.F. Mime Troupe, Morgan Upton of The Committee, photographer Robert Altman, astrologer Barbara Birdfeather, *Rag*'s writer Larieta Merrick, Cherubic Rona Elliot and 85 other equally zany characters. (These names are given for the convenience of U.S. Army intelligence officers who collect such information.) Kineticolor's Dick Rosenblatt, who was responsible for this surrealistic scene, beamed from his seat, almost at ease. The plane taxied to the runway, revved its motors and took off to thunderous applause. Immediately, joints appeared and were passed through the plane.

As soon as the "Fasten Seat Belts" sign flashed off, Ricki Stein, recently returned from the Pit River Indians sortie, lurched down the aisle playing rock music from a cassette through a bullhorn, a blur of wild hair, beard and Indian sari. Meals were served by the stewardesses, only one of whom was tight-lipped and tight-assed. The others were stoned from breathing the cabin air.

Soon we were discussing the mysterious conference and

weaving fantasies/paranoid ideation. How about a New York *Times* headline reading "Tragic Air Explosion Wipes Out Underground Media," I suggest to Krassner. He came back with "Oh, no, 'Tragic' would be editorializing."

Another theory was that the plane hadn't really taken off but was in a hangar with scenes of clouds and sky flashing on the hangar walls. Soon the gas jets would be turned on and . . .

Or when the plane refueled in Des Moines (we had a relatively small 3-engine jet) we'd be loaded into buses and driven to the camps. . . .

The most popular idea was a hijacking to Cuba, especially since no one on the plane would have protested. But one person would have had to remain behind in Cuba and no one wanted to volunteer. So the ideas and champagne flowed and the plane and its merry cargo got higher and higher. We hoped the pilot didn't share our air supply.

The vibes were so good on the plane that Mr. Wiggins, United's beefy-faced passenger service agent, was moved to announce over the P.A. system that contrary to all expectations he had enjoyed the flight immensely and looked forward to the return flight. So did we.

For hours we watched a thunderstorm to starboard, lightning backlighting cloud formations, a fantastic light show.

Scene: 3 A.M. at the Burlington, Vermont, airport. We exit the plane through the tail to thunderous applause—from us. For as we reach the ground we turn and applaud and cheer each passenger.

Larry Yurden, Goddard College alumnus, perpetually five o'clock shadowed and fatigued originator and chief conspirator of the Alternative Media Conference, greets us and directs the freak show to waiting Greyhound buses. Another improbable character directly out of R. Crumb's imagination, delivers a check for $17,000 to the pilot and we're off.

An hour or so later in the wet predawn light we tumble from the buses into a cafeteria where we're assigned rooms and keys and schedules and maps and suddenly it seems like summer camp. That's what it's all about, some kind of P.A.L. summer camp for depra(i)ved media freaks, or is it? We trundle off to the dorms through beautiful bountiful Vermont woods, I with a new Pisces lady wondering why lately I have been swimming around with so many foxy fishes. She knows me fairly well already, this little one, since she is deeply into astrology and naturally knows our sign best and I coincidentally (maybe) have many of its characteristics.

We stow our gear in dormitory rooms and walk through the Goddard campus. Signs point to the campgrounds. Signs like "Sunshine—this way" or "Please don't feed the bears acid."

Stoned humor but someone has organized this trip extremely well. In the early morning mist we see a few funky schoolbuses, tents, people in sleeping bags, VW pop-up campers. The Hog Farm has yet to arrive.

On another road we two sit on a log, feeling the greenness, listening to bullfrogs, wondering how they make the sounds they do—like plucked inch-wide bass strings. You see, this all is very relevant to the Alternative Media Conference. Goddard College was the setting. We brought our sets. Just up the hill from our log was the new library where in the next few days the alternative media had the best view of itself.

Okay, let's flash briefly to the library well Wednesday night. Bob Fass of New York's WBAI is conducting a workshop billed as "Free Enterprise and the Cultural Revolution," except it's really a wild Bob Fass mixed-media trip. John Shules is trying to say some words on behalf of Holding Together and Tim Leary who's been in jail since . . . WHAT ABOUT BOBBY SEALE? someone screams, HE'S BEEN JAIL SINCE . . . Fass is drowned out too. There's a guy in a beret and uniform, waving a gun. Everyone is yelling, cursing, screaming when suddenly Morgan Upton thunders out the clearest, truest message, FREE THE INDIANAPOLIS 500, and disappears into the night.

At the same time four other workshops as well as a square dance and films are scattered over the campus. One of the films is *Taos, Love and Peace, 1970.*

Thursday Morning

Sleepy people ghost-walking on a cafeteria line. Remarkably cheerful Goddard College students serving up good old homemade crunchy granola and French toast. Sliding the tray along I see a plate labeled something like "Dope Gratefully Accepted." A joint on the plate soon has lots of company. No dope paranoia at Goddard. Vermonters won't bother you if you don't bother them.

Morning workshops—seven are scheduled. "Pirate and Guerrilla Radio" looks interesting. Visions of offshore transmitters and black vans hurtling through city streets broadcasting cryptic messages like "This is your new Mayor-President-Dictator speaking."

Another was "Radio Drama (Remember It?)" and I could almost hear the "Lux Radio Theater," "The Shadow," "Inner Sanctum," "I Love A Mystery" . . .

But I went to "Public Affairs" conducted by Scoop Nisker and Larry Bensky because I'd heard them on San Francisco's KSAN doing their news collages, liking most of them, hating some of them. Scoop played some of his famous tapes, like the one which begins with Nixon's voice saying, "We are not invading Cambodia" . . . They're on a record now. There was lots of talk in the room from other participants about "when we take over" . . . "we'll off them then" . . . and other power games. They spat out the words *peace* and *love*. While Joshua of San Francisco's KMPX played an ecology tape, cigarette butts were thrown out the window.

By that time the lines were being drawn. There were media people, movement people and movement people in the media and little agreement among the groups. My question of "What is news?" was met with silence.

Jerry Rubin made a brief appearance. We saw each other in the cafeteria and turned away. Later I was pissed at myself for allowing politics to prevent human greetings. A story circulated that evening that Nancy Rubin's wallet containing $500 had been ripped off. The Conference paid them $250 and they left in a cloud of ill will.

A conference of "Humor" conducted by Marshall Efrom soon turned into a vituperative series of arguments led largely by Ronnie Davis. Several people present showed their disgust by bending over and baring their bottoms.

Meanwhile, on the campus . . . people swam nude in the pond while bongo drummers laid out a stoned beat. Bands played on an outdoor stage, polyethylene air structures sprang up in the woods, the Hog Farm fed people from a huge tent, new video techniques were demonstrated by groups like Videofreex, people walking through the woods suddenly heard Tim Leary's recorded voice booming out, "Live and let live . . ."

Friday

I slept through the morning conferences. One of them was "Drugs and the Media." When I went outside I saw hundreds of people with orange spots placed on their noses by the Hog Farm. Marked for safety while tripping. No bad trips were reported, at least none that required medical treatment. Many people wandering in the woods or lying on the ground looking at flowers or blades of grass. The tabs were said to be Sunshine. Dr. John played till four A.M. in the Haybarn Theater.

The day before, Morgan, Larie and I had watched three little girls 8 or 9 years old playing in the empty theater. They had worked up a routine which they called "The Three Chicks" and it was a pretty good act. Larie and I saw the girls later that day skipping down the road to Plainfield, the town just outside the campus limits. We had just met Parker, a young bearded reporter for the *Boston Globe*, their "token hippie" as he put it. Parker was glum because one of his weekly columns had been axed by the *Globe*.

"What was it about?" I asked. He told me the column

concerned Dr. Pusey, Harvard's outgoing president, who had recently made a speech comparing some of the New Left to Joseph McCarthy. Pusey was one of the few brave enough to speak out against McCarthyism during the time students were known as the Silent Generation (when Nixon played the same heavy role he gave to Agnew).

"Don't you think the comparison has some validity?" I asked. "The students Pusey refers to don't have the power of government behind them but they feel exactly the same way Joseph McCarthy did about free speech."

Parker then related a story about the editors and staff of the Boston University newspaper being beaten in their offices for printing a story critical of Women's Liberation. He didn't feel too good about the incident. I remembered the time when the staff of the San Francisco State newspaper was attacked. I remembered the bombings of the *Los Angeles Free Press* and the attempted firebombing of the *Berkeley Barb*. "It's the same old shit whether the attacks come from the right or left, Parker. Free speech is a precious right. Maybe the Alternative Media will take a good look at itself during this conference and learn something." But I was sorry his column had been axed.

Saturday

The library well again. A workshop on "Comics and Mass Consciousness" with Harvey Kurtzman, Stan Lee and Marc Estrin. Suddenly several couples wrapped in blankets appear. They lie on the floor and begin to fuck. Instant chaos. On the other side of the room members of a women's liberation group are screaming and clawing at the faces of their opponents, while the others in the room can only gape at the scene around them. The Alternative Media conference officially ends.

Saturday Night

The California contingent remains on campus waiting for our plane which will arrive the following night. We're in love with Vermont and some of us decide not to return.

Small parties in the dorms. Lots of dope smoked. Campus security guards and sheriff's deputies wander through glancing at the dope smokers. No hassles.

"Hey!" one bright young guy says, "almost all the underground media was represented here. We could create any myths we want!"

"Hey," I said, "there was another guy who thought the same thing, name of Goebbels."

They passed a hash pipe round and round until even our bright young friend was mellow.

Sunday

Lazy day. No workshops, Pisces lady and I hitchhike to Barre, "the granite city." Everything made of granite there. Granite post office, granite tombstone company, Granite Insurance Company. We stop at Dunkin Doughnuts which are soft and bad for us but taste so good. "Forgive me, J. I. Rodale," I mutter as I do myself in with a blueberry doughnut. We buy two dozen more for our friends and hitchhike back, picked up by a kid in a Rambler who lives in Plainfield and once got as far west as Oklahoma. He tells us of Vermont winters and snowmobiles roaring through frozen fields. And we're sorry we must leave Vermont.

Sunday Night

Burlington airport. Twenty empty seats for the flight to California and twenty-six hitchhikers. Hiding in the johns and in front of the seats most plan to fly to the coast and hitchhike back. At first it's funny but it goes on and on and on. There's so little baggage everyone knows there's no weight problem but FAA regulations say no more than 96 people may fly. So it's on again and off again and finally lots are drawn and six are left behind in Burlington. And then we discover two more empty seats. With a mighty Om we lift the plane from the runway. Off goes the "Fasten Seat Belts" sign. On goes the P.A. "A hash pipe is urgently needed in the forward cabin."

I'm asked to read some letters so grab the P.A. "This

is Henrique Fernandez your new captain speaking." I'm not about to mention anything like Cuba even in jest. Not when Peter Townsend is hassled by the F.B.I. for saying one of the WHO records "bombed." I read a letter about "Pixie dust"—mint leaves soaked in PCP, an animal tranquilizer. "Where can I get some?" someone yells.

Next a letter from a girl suffering from painful intercourse. "It's better to have had dyspareunia than no pareunia," I begin and then am cut off by the real captain. "He has an eighteen-year-old daughter," explains a stewardess.

We land in Des Moines and Scoop leaves the plane, off to visit family in Minneapolis. We can't leave even for a few minutes because on the flight east we danced on the runway, freaking the service employees.

The rest of the trip is subdued and we have dawn for hours before sighting San Francisco. Remembering a promise to write about the flight home and wanting to write about something new to me, lady friend and I lock ourselves into a john intending to truly fly United but it's too funny and too contrived so we don't. In the never-to-be-published *Realist* Tenth Anniversary issue, Paul has me balling Dear Abby which I might try if only she'd fly United with me. And then we are down. Mr. Wiggins asks us to check the aircraft, emphasizing nothing should be left behind. We go to the baggage area and then farewell for now to Pisces lady, farewell for a while to my media friends. We feel more together than when we left, individually and collectively. We are one.

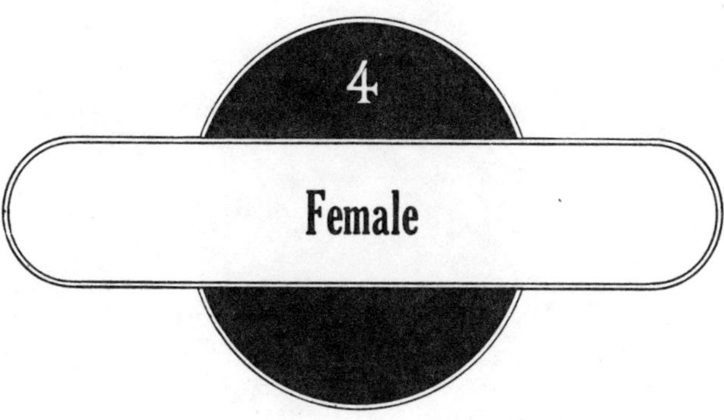

4
Female

Her First Pelvic Exam

"My first year at Stephens College all the girls were getting weird diseases. They were just starting to make it with boys and went to the college dispensary with a whole lot of vaginal complaints—trichomonas, fungus infections and strange discharges that didn't seem to have a name."

My laboratory assistant and I were discussing the ways emotional distress is often expressed through bodily complaints. In females, distress is often literally discharged through the vagina. Gynecologists are all too familiar with stubborn vaginal infections that clear up only when the patient's mental state improves.

"I'll never forget my first gynecologic examination. I was really scared. Getting undressed wasn't so bad. Then I lay down on the examining table and the nurse put my feet in those metal things, what are they called?"

"Stirrups. They're to hold your legs up, apart and steady so the doctor can see everything he has to see."

"One of my girlfriends said she was examined by a doctor who didn't have a nurse in the room. I thought that was a law."

"There's no such law. The nurse is there to hand instruments to the doctor and also to protect him from the possibility of a rape charge."

"So there's no such law?"

"No. And I think some women would be more comfortable if only the doctor were there, though, of course, others feel better if a nurse is in the room. Doctors are considered good targets by some predatory patients and lawyers who know they are forced to carry malpractice insurance in large sums."

"Well, then the nurse hung a sheet over my legs. What's that for?"

"Some women get nervous when they see the doctor exploring their private parts. It's also less embarrassing for those who would be embarrassed—both doctor and patient."

"First, he seemed to be examining the outside of me. What was he doing?"

"He was examining the entrance to the vagina, the Bartholin glands which secrete lubricating fluid, the urethra and the clitoris."

"Then he used one of those instruments that are always so COLD!"

"That was a speculum. They're made of stainless steel and look something like a duck's bill. Many doctors try to warm them before use so they're less uncomfortable."

"What's it used for?"

"With a speculum a doctor can see the inside of the vagina including the cervix. First he lubricates the two rounded blades of the speculum so it's easier to insert. After it's in the vagina, he can spread the blades by pushing a lever. If there's a discharge, he'll note the color and odor and can take part of it for laboratory examination. Usually he'll do a Pap smear too."

"A Pap smear is a cancer test, isn't it?"

"Yup. There's always some discharge even in a healthy vagina. Some of this mucus as well as a smear of the cervix is taken for microscopic examination. Very early cancer can first be picked up by examination of cells which have been sloughed from the cancerous tissue."

She shuddered, "I don't think I want any more Pap smears. It'd be horrible to find out I had cancer."

"Not at all. Cancer of the cervix in that stage is 100 percent curable."

"Anyway, that metal thing, besides being cold, is so hard. It hurts. Why don't they make them softer—like bodies." Her green eyes twinkled a bit.

"Well, they have to be sterilized for one thing. And I

think that even if they were body soft (or hard) there would still be complaints of pain because many women are literally up-tight during a gynecologic exam. Plastic specula are available. That would solve the cold problem but they break easily and can be used only once so they're comparatively expensive."

"Because it was my first pelvic exam, the doctor decided to tell me about everything he was doing. After he finished the speculum examination, he examined me with his hands."

"A doctor's hands are among his most sensitive instruments. Part of a gynecologic examination includes palpating or feeling the internal organs of reproduction—the uterus, Fallopian tubes and ovaries."

"That's right," she said, "he would push up from inside me and have me feel just above the pubis with my hand whatever he was examining."

" 'Do you know what this is?' he would ask.

" 'No, what is it?'

" 'That's your right ovary.'

"He did that with both ovaries, tubes and my uterus. After a while, I wasn't scared at all. I was mostly curious about what I was going to feel next. Finally he pushed up from inside again. 'What's that? What's that?' I was really curious.

" 'That's my right index finger,' he said."

Obscenity or Information?

The "school kids" issue of England's underground newspaper *Oz* led to an infamous obscenity trial ending with the editors sentenced to long prison terms. A Hip Pocrates column was part of the evidence. Later, the convictions were overturned and the net result was a tremendous increase in *Oz*'s circulation.

But the column alone has caused legal problems to only one newspaper, so far as I know, Vancouver, B.C.'s *Georgia Straight*. One of the oldest and best of the undergrounds, the *Georgia Straight* is edited by Dan McLeod, a quiet but very strong-willed Canadian. Dan has persevered despite years of police harassment and lack of support from Vancouver's staid dailies. One of the *Straight*'s many police busts involved a classified ad using the term "muff-diver" (ancient slang for cunnilingus). A comical trial followed but judgment was held in abeyance. The Vancouver police then read each *Georgia Straight* issue, word for word, waiting for another chance to shut down the newspaper.

The following letter began a series of legal maneuvers which led to my first visit to Vancouver:

Dear Dr. Schoenfeld:

This is extremely important to me. I am 17 years old and I have pills so I won't get pregnant.

The problem is that I have slept with boys but never had intercourse because it has hurt too much. Is there anything at all I can do to lessen the pain? I am open to all suggestions.

P.S. I am not sleeping around carelessly. I have been going with my boyfriend for seven months.

ANSWER: I think you should have a gynecological examination to determine whether there is a physical basis for the pain you feel. My laboratory assistant suggests that barring any physical problem the pain will turn to pleasure if you are free of guilt and find someone you love.

The medical term for painful intercourse is dyspareunia. One of my medical school classmates used to say, "It's better to have dyspareunia than no pareunia at all." But he didn't have dyspareunia.

My answer apparently wasn't specific enough for I received a letter with direct instructions which were published exactly as received:

"A while back a girl wrote in to you, asking what to do about her problem of severe pain during intercourse. Having been through this same problem myself I felt that your advice was singularly unhelpful, and finally decided to send some of my own along.

1. *Lubricate well as you can. Getting your boyfriend to eat you is a good idea.*
2. *Take it* slowly. *Ease the cock in at* your *desired speed. Don't let anyone push you faster than you want to go at any time.*
3. *Keep your legs fairly wide apart, but not to a point where it is a strain to keep them there.*
4. *Relax. Relax. Relax. Sometimes this may mean thinking about something besides sex and what's happening at the moment.*
5. *Part of it is just time, waiting till you get stretched out enough (or whatever happens). And Really, it does happen at last."*

When the letter was printed, Vancouver police seized 2000 copies of the *Georgia Straight*, arrested Dan McLeod and charged him with four counts of obscenity including publishing obscenity for profit, a charge I found amusing since the straits of the *Straight* hadn't permitted payment for my column for 18 months. A rock benefit was planned with Country Joe McDonald and Barry Melton. Would I read some letters? Sure. So early one foggy Berkeley morning I waited on the corner of Russell and Ellsworth for a ride to the airport. We were late for our Canadian Pacific plane and raced into the terminal. C.P. ticket agents saw us running toward the counter and pointed to the correct gate. We were the last passengers.

The customs officials in Vancouver seemed to know who we were but they waved Barry and me through the lines.

Joe had recently been busted and his luggage was thoroughly inspected. Naturally we carried no contraband.

That night there was a large crowd for the benefit. After Barry and Joe sang, I read letters which seemed interesting to me, including the one causing the bust. I thought I might be busted also but no hassles arose and several thousand dollars were raised for legal costs.

The trial was held several months later. Witnesses for the defense included myself, a Canadian physician and a housewife. I donned the first tie I'd worn in years and gave my background and reasons for including the letter. The other physician testified that the advice given was useful and valid. I think the most important testimony came from the young married woman who stated she had been troubled by dyspareunia and was helped by the column. Charges were eventually dismissed.

Masturbation Guilt

Dear Dr. Hip Pocrates:

I am 15 years old and am a girl. I have been masturbating (just recently finding out the name of it) for three years. Is this normal?

I don't think my friends do it—that's why I'm worried. The reason I think my friends don't do it is because they seem more . . . well, immature than me. They like Walt Disney movies and won't kiss their boyfriends. They are happier than I am.

Sometimes I go for a couple of months without doing it, but then all of a sudden I am doing it once a day for a week. I think it happens mostly when I am lonely or depressed. Is there any way of getting over this?

P.S. Thank you for reading this; for taking the time to read it. Even if you don't answer, it's a relief for me to tell someone.

ANSWER: In *Human Sexual Response*, Masters and Johnson report that, physiologically, an "orgasm is an orgasm," however it is achieved. But most people find greater satisfaction when sex is shared with another person.

"I don't care what Masters and Johnson found in their research," my secretary wisely pointed out, tapping her head, "it's up here that counts."

Dear Dr. Schoenfeld:

I have an awful problem. I am an 18-year-old female, fairly pretty, and have no problem getting nice (or the right) guys. Right now I have a special man whom I love dearly. We are planning to be married, and there is nothing for which I could hope for more. But even marriage will leave me, quite literally, "frustrated."

When I was a very young girl, maybe four or five, I discovered masturbation. It seemed to please me; yet I had no idea what it was or if it was wrong or right. I always achieved orgasm. I had a climax by laying on a table, balancing on the corner, where my organs rested (now that I write this out, in plain English, it seems perfectly awful).

My parents never told me about sex. I was quite naive until the end of 10th grade, which is rather late, I am sure. My mother won't discuss S-E-X with me, since it's a dirty word. My stepfather found pleasure in doing sexual things with me forcefully.

My problem is this: I cannot achieve orgasm now, nor anything like it. I cry at night, knowing that although I satisfy my guy, he falsely thinks he is satisfying me. Sometimes, though rarely, he doubts whether he satisfies me or not, and maybe he wonders if he is acting right. I can't discuss this problem with him. How could it help to let the facts be known? He would then consider having sex with me to be selfish.

Continuing the cause of the problem: until 7th or 8th grade, I could achieve orgasm. What I must have done is damaged the nerves, since my clitoris seems nonexistent. I got so frustrated when I could not achieve climax, even by masturbation, that I often felt so depressed I saw no reason to live. It made me, and still makes me feel like an unwhole person.

I don't think that my stepfather's attacks have made my mind closed to the mental side of sex. I am quite sure it is physical.

It makes me so happy to see my boyfriend reach climax. It makes me so happy, I can't let you know how much. Yet I do feel a little jealous. It's like he can have me, but I can't have him. I think that my jealousy is justified, too. Sex is sharing when people are in love.

ANSWER: Masturbation hasn't rotted your brain or your clitoris. But guilt over masturbation still causes great misery even though it's a normal means of sexual release practiced by most women and almost all men sometime in their lives or perhaps all through life. The method you described as "awful" is commonly used by females, though softer objects, like pillows, are usually employed.

Difficulty in achieving orgasm is a common problem in females. There is no one common answer except that physical causes for this complaint are extremely rare. The best solution for you might be to consult with a qualified marriage counselor. Your local health department should be able to make such a referral. Other sources of information are free clinics (which usually have privately practicing therapists on their staffs) or psychiatric and counseling clinics of nearby universities.

The Clitoris

What's in a Name?

Dear Dr. Schoenfeld:

Could you please tell me if there is any other word for "clitoris"? That's just too scientifically proper for bedroom talk, but neither my boyfriend nor any of my other friends have been able to find one that seems natural to say.

We agree that "clit" is only a little bit better so your suggestions really will be appreciated.

ANSWER: Three syllables does seem out of proportion but I've never heard another word for this unique organ which has pleasure as its only known function. Perhaps there are readers with other suggestions.

"A clitoris could only be called fanciful names of a nonmedical flavor such as 'touch me often,' 'joyspot' or 'Love's dimple.' "

"Tickler" (from San Francisco's Rev. Jefferson Fuck Poland).

"I think the slang dictionaries may list a few terms such as 'bean' and 'the little man in the boat'—pretty unattractive. How about 'panic button.' "

From someone in Berkeley who calls himself The Red Ant:

"Perhaps the Mexicans have a good idea; they call it 'la lenguita,' or 'the little tongue.' "

Dear Dr. Schoenfeld:

In the Name-the-Clit sweepstakes, one dare not overlook the unsolicited contribution proffered by Lennon and McCartney in the lyrics of "Happiness Is a Warm Gun," i.e. "trigger."

Inasmuch as stimulation of the clitoral switch inclines one to become turned on (and turns one on to becoming inclined), we might say that it is the "toggle" which we tickle. Since this clit is located in the box-top, how's about "Cupid's coupon." Or, to mint a phrase: "bille-doux"—literally, "sweet little nut." Not to be confused with "billet-doux," which is a love note, not a love node.

"Love bead?" Love-bud? Hump-bump? Or the succulent Elizabethan metaphor: the pearl? To a cunnilingophile, a "lollypop." To the swinger, "a local fun spot."

And to each, his own.

Hooded Clitoris?

Dear Dr. Schoenfeld:

I am a single girl of 23 who has a most frustrating problem—I am unable to reach a climax (except through cunnilingus or masturbation) because I have a hooded clitoris.

I know there is an operation to remove the hood, but I am also sure I could not afford it. Therefore, I write to you to ask if you might know of any positions that would help me reach a climax.

I have tried all the well-known positions (and other types too) but I'll be damned if I can ever climax through intercourse!

ANSWER: I doubt that a "hooded" clitoris is the cause of your complaint or that surgery would be helpful.

Some sex therapists use a conditioning technique for women able to climax through masturbation or manipulation by her partner, but not with vaginal intercourse. First, she is brought to orgasm by her partner's fingers, he facing her rear with his penis at the entrance to her vagina. Over a period of several weeks she is brought to orgasm during full penile penetration. Patience and perfect frankness between partners is necessary for this treatment to be effective.

Electric vibrators are recommended by many gynecologists to women with orgasmic difficulties. Some females unable to climax through masturbation, oral sex, or a partner's digital manipulations, have reached orgasm the first time with a vibrator. The fear that a vibrator will become the only possible means of satisfaction does not seem often justified. Battery-operated vibrators are usually too weak to be effective, despite their phallic shapes.

Virginity

Stretching the Hymen

Dear Dr. Schoenfeld:

I'm going with this guy who's 18 and I'm 15. We have been going together for 2 months and sex is normal in a relationship such as this.

He told me if I don't want to have sex that he loves me enough to go along with this (we have been having it once in a while). But what I want to know is when he touches me is there any chance of me losing my virginity in any way by stretching or tearing of my hymen?

I know I should know this and really aren't this dumb but this is very important to me and our relationship.

ANSWER: If your friend knows his (or rather your) anatomy the hymen needn't be touched. Otherwise it might very well be stretched or torn. Hymens are frequently torn anyway through childhood accidents.

Menstruation in Virgins

Dear Dr. Schoenfeld:

If a girl's hymen is intact, how does the menstrual blood get out?

ANSWER: Only rarely does the hymen completely cover the vaginal opening. One or more small openings permit flow of menstrual blood.

Cyclic pain and cramping without bleeding in a young girl may indicate an imperforate hymen. Prompt medical attention is then necessary to prevent serious consequences.

Virgin Questions

Dear Dr. Schoenfeld:

I am a 13-year-old chick, who 4 days ago, lost my virginity. The dude I balled and I were very drunk and I didn't come. He seemed to come very well though. What could have caused this?

This guy has had a lot of chicks. I have been assured by 2 of this dude's close friends and one of his old girlfriends that he doesn't have clap, and I believe them. Do you think I should get a VD test?

ANSWER: You seem to understand that the more sexual contacts a person has, the greater the chance of getting a venereal disease. But your friend doesn't necessarily have gonorrhea or syphilis. If he knew he had a venereal disease and cared about you he would let you know right away. But rather than worry, you can visit the free VD clinic of your local health department.

You didn't say whether you or he had used a contraceptive. Planned Parenthood has classes and clinics which could be very helpful.

Guys usually don't have trouble reaching an orgasm when they're with a girl for the first time—but it's more difficult for girls.

Bleeding

Normal Bleeding

Dear Dr. Schoenfeld:

I have a problem which is embarrassing and troublesome to me. A few weeks ago, I balled for the first time (incidentally, I'm a girl) and bled an awful lot.

I would like to know: Is the bleeding just because it was the first time? Or is there something wrong with me?

If not, could you tell me how to stop the bleeding? I'm sort of doubtful about doing it again until I have an answer.

ANSWER: There's no doubt at all you should learn more about your own body, and soon. Bleeding is normal in a female the first few times she has sexual intercourse. The cause is tearing or stretching of the hymen, a tissue membrane nearly covering the entrance to the vagina.

Many girls are free of bleeding and pain even the first time they have sexual intercourse. Their hymens may have been stretched or torn by exercise or childhood accidents. Some women, though, have hymenal tissue so tough that minor surgery is required before normal relations can begin.

You should soon have a thorough pelvic examination and discussion with a physician about ways to prevent pregnancy.

Abnormal Bleeding

Dear Dr. Schoenfeld:

Everytime me and my boyfriend have intercourse, I always bleed a lot. It gets to be a real hangup because there is an awful lot of blood which gets all over the sheets, etc.

None of my other girlfriends have this problem and I was wondering if something could be wrong with me. Or is this normal in some people? Please advise because I'm worried.

ANSWER: A gynecologic examination should determine the cause of this abnormal bleeding. Don't delay seeing your family doctor or a gynecologist. Your county medical association or nearest medical school can recommend a physician or clinic in your area.

Survival

Dear Dr. Schoenfeld:

I am a college co-ed, and I belong to a group which will soon embark on a long survival hike.

I have already given up cosmetics and have had my hair cut extremely short. Now my only problem is what to do about menstruation.

This is of some concern to me, because no one has any idea as to how long the trip will last (although we are all taking this semester and next off for it), and I am allowed to bring only as much equipment as I can carry in a backpack. I am wondering whether to go on the Pill.

ANSWER: Birth control pills should not be used to postpone menstruation. Compact tampons are available and a supply of several months would occupy little space in your backpack. Before disposable napkins and tampons were available women used soft washable pieces of cloth. If you'll be away indefinitely that might be best for you though not very convenient.

Dear Dr. Schoenfeld:

Your correspondent who needs a way to backpack menstrual supplies might find very useful the small collapsible plastic cups that fit within the vagina and have a triple leakproof seal. True, they are a little bulkier and trickier to use than tampons, but enough better to be worth the effort. A girl with a tight hymen might experience some pain, especially on removal, but it's my opinion that, if so, she ought to persevere or she'll have one helluva wedding night.

Of course, the manufacturer recommends flushing them away. But they aren't biodegradable and concern for our poor abused ocean led me to discover that they can be very easily and quickly washed and reinserted. They require changing only every 12 to 24 hours and so half a dozen of them should last our backpacker almost indefinitely. Check them out at a pharmacy or supermarket.

Female M.D.

Absent Menses

Dear Dr. Schoenfeld:

I am a 15-year-old girl with an apparent problem. Three years ago I began having my period which continued fairly regularly for almost two years. For the last year I haven't had it at all.

I have never had sexual intercourse so I could not be pregnant.

ANSWER: Menstrual irregularities are common during adolescence and often girls will go for months without a period. But a year is a long time so I would advise you to consult a gynecologist soon.

By the way, several pregnancies in virgins have been verified in recent times. They occurred when semen was ejaculated near the vaginal opening.

Vaginal Discharges

Embarrassed

Dear Dr. Hip Pocrates:

I know the latest trend is to go without underwear, but even with my modest length skirts I wouldn't dare. My vagina constantly drips a milky substance. I am pretty sure it isn't a discharge of disease, because it is not discolored, doesn't itch, and I have had it for years. In the last few years this drip has become more of a problem.

Since I don't plan to go around without underwear, I am not worried about leaving a trail like Hansel & Gretel, but I don't like my underwear to look dirty after two or three hours. Sometimes my boyfriend will take off some of my clothes and it embarrasses me to think he might notice.

I think the drip is the result of sexual arousal, but since I don't think I'm abnormally preoccupied with sex, I wonder what to do.

This is really too embarrassing to mention to my gynecologist.

ANSWER: Chronic sexual arousal is, unfortunately, the least likely source of a chronic vaginal discharge. Common causes are trichomonas, fungal and gonorrheal infections, erosion of the cervix or a reaction to birth control pills. Your gynecologist will neither be shocked by your questions nor embarrass you with his answers.

Dear Dr. Schoenfeld:

Regarding the letter from the girl who complained of a "vaginal drip." I think if her boyfriend notices, it could be one of the best things that ever happened to him (at least that's the way I feel about honey).

Neither my girlfriend nor I feel any embarrassment over her constant "wetness."

ANSWER: Constant "wetness" may be normal or could indicate a vaginal infection. Discharges from vaginitis can dampen a girl's ardor.

Unfeminine Hygiene

The Medical Letter is a scientific newsletter which evaluates drugs and chemical products. A full page of the October 16, 1970, issue was devoted to feminine hygiene deodorant sprays. They began investigating these products after receiving reports of inflammatory reactions and rashes in the vulvo-vaginal areas. The first thing they learned is that the manufacturers of these sprays "are not required to provide proof of their safety or usefulness or to reveal their chemical contents." The manufacturers were reluctant to disclose this information.

Medical Letter's conclusion is as follows: "It is unlikely that commercial deodorant feminine hygiene sprays are as effective as soap and water in promoting a hygienic and odor-free external genital surface."

Dr. Bernard Kaye, an Illinois obstetrician-gynecologist, wrote a letter to the *Journal of the A.M.A.* warning against these useless sprays saying ". . . good old-fashioned soap and water should do the same thing. I have cautioned my patients not to use these sprays and recommend that other physicians do likewise."

Yeast Infections

Dear Dr. Schoenfeld:

I've just been to a doctor who says I have monilia (yeast) infection. He prescribed suppositories and said not to fuck for 15 days.

He also said the male is not a carrier so my husband doesn't need to be treated. My questions are:

1) *If the male isn't a carrier why can't I fuck for 15 days if my cunt feels up to it and, most importantly*
2) *If the male isn't a carrier how did I get this disease? It seems very coincidental that I got this (never had it before) after sexual contact with a person whose old lady had it too.*

I really need some answers because me and my old man are getting into a group marriage relationship with the couple I just mentioned and we need to know who can fuck with whom when one of the females has monilia (or trichomonas). For instance, can my old man be with the other old lady without giving monilia back to her?

ANSWER: Most physicians believe yeast infections are not transferred through sexual contact—that's the way it's taught in medical school. But other physicians, including myself, think monilial infections can be transmitted this way.

Thrush infections (a monilial infection of the mouth) in newborn babies, for example, often result from contact with the infected mother during childbirth.

Uncircumcised males are more likely to harbor yeast organisms than those who are circumcised, but in any case, proper personal hygiene should reduce the possibility of transmitting the disease. The reason for abstaining from sexual intercourse while your infection is under treatment is to prevent further irritation of the inflamed tissues.

Yeasty Group

Dear Dr. Schoenfeld:

This letter is in response to the woman with a vaginal yeast infection who is entering a group marriage.

We established a group marriage 2½ years ago and the wives suffered from yeast infections for at least a year thereafter. My mother would suggest God was getting his revenge on us for being so sinful. At this time there seems to be no problem and so I believe we have all gotten used to each other's bugs.

But the head problems turned out to be a lot heavier than the body problems and we have spent a good deal of bread on therapy.

Yeast Cure Uncovered

FLASH! A Berkeley physician has cleared up recurrent vaginal yeast infections in his patients by suggesting they stop wearing underpants. Yeast infections plague many women, especially those who take birth control pills or antibiotics. These medications alter the normal ecology of the vagina, permitting yeast organisms to grow in great numbers. Leather pants or any other tight-fitting, relatively impermeable garments favor the proliferation of the yeast, which grows best in a warm moist environment. Nylon panties, then, should not be worn by women with recurrent monilial infections.

My secretary recommends panty slips to prevent cold bottoms or embarrassment when wearing short skirts. Or if the idea still chills you, wear cotton panties.

Dear Dr. Schoenfeld:

I am in excellent health but was annoyed with excessive vaginal moistness and an unpleasant odor. Took your ad-

vice—changed from nylon panties to cotton panties three weeks ago, and the problem is solved. Thank you.

Old Wives' Tale

Dear Dr. Hip:

PANTY SCANTY! My heavens! Shuffle off to Buffalo, as we used to say (long ago). You doctors are going to be but nowhere until you break down and put an official OLD WIFE on the staff of your medical schools.

Here's how to REALLY cure up the itch:

a) *Send away everybody in the house.*
b) *Take a nice warm shower—or any kind of shower. Douche with clear water. CLEAR WATER. While you are in the shower. Get out. Dry off.*
c) *Lie down on your back in front of a forced warm air heater. Summertime? Use a fan.*
d) *Bend your knees up. Manipulate your abdomen, arse, leg and thigh muscles up, down, tight, loose, any which way you can think of UNTIL YOU CAN HEAR AND FEEL AIR MOVING IN AND OUT OF YOUR VAGINA. If you can't hear it whooshing in and out you aren't doing it right.*
e) *When you have had enough lying around on the floor whooshing and thinking, get up and go to work. Do this once or twice a day until the itch goes away. THAT'S IT.*

Will she stay cured? If she reinfects, another treatment is as cheap and close as her nearest shower and heater and fan.

Naturally I do not charge for this advice. The neat thing about OLD WIVES is that they NEVER charge (professional ethics).

I even throw in a bit more good advice: I always have my girls begin by jumping rope 100 times—before the shower bit. This does not do anything for the itch, BUT I DON'T TELL THEM THAT. It is great for knocking off a few pounds and tightening up a few muscles. By the time the itch is gone they are firm from waist to tippy toe and look like the most! *If you don't look THE MOST, you might as well have the itch, I always say.*

Sincerely yours,
Old (but very slim) Wife

Dear Doc:

The Old Wife who wrote to you was right if the "itch" she spoke about was the common yeast infection or Vaginitis. (Boy—do I know about those!)

You get all kinds of itching and a cheesy discharge. The doctor will usually give you tablets to schtoop up your vagina but the best thing is warm air and lots of it. Avoid baths—showers are best. My doctor advised me to lay down, spread my legs and sun with a heat lamp for a short time. "Don't wear panties," he said.

The Old Wife's cure may not be good for gonorrhea but it's great for this one!

Love and Peace

Hoo! Hoo!

Dear Dr. Schoenfeld:

One major cause of chronic yeast infections is the ultra cleanliness hang-up of using Phisohex (hexachlorophene) or deodorant soaps to scrupulously scrub the female genitalia.*

I, too, was guilty of this with resultant itch and irritation until my friendly GYN man pointed out the obvious—these marvelous bug killers also *do in the good bacteria which control the yeast: voila! the itch!*

I am an R.N. who has told quite a few girls about this and they find that in a week or less the problem no longer exists.

In other words, girls, don't be quite so fanatical about a smidgen of natural scent of female. Scrub the rest of your

* Note: hexachlorophene is now available only by doctor's prescription.

body with all the deodorant soaps you want to, but for crying out loud use baby or some other mild soap for your hoo-hoo.

V.C.

Dear Dr.,

As president of a local Hoo-Hoo-Ette club, and a director of the National Hoo-Hoo-Ettes, I would like to comment on the letter from the R.N.

Hoo-Hoo-Ettes is a National Organization of women employed in the forest and lumber products industries, and related fields. V.C. does not know what a hoo-hoo is, but it is certainly not what she said to wash with mild soap.

Your column was read aloud, with much delight, at the National Board Meeting in Los Angeles on Saturday, February 20, [1971]. Thank you for affording a little more humor to a very busy meeting.

Sincerely,
Jane Carpenter, President
Tehama County Hoo-Hoo-Ettes #15

Opposite Cure—Same Result

Dear Dr. Schoenfeld:

A last word on yeast infections. You are wasting your time talking about cotton underwear. The answer is Phiso-hex!

Used regularly, this has prevented any yeast infections for me for a year and a half—and I used to get them every other month for a decade. Actually, I recently got one again, the direct result of an increased sex life.

So I can only conclude that if you've tried everything else—a yeast infection is nature's way of telling you to slow down.

ANSWER: I can only conclude that yeast infections often respond to positive suggestions.

What's Your Type?

Dear Dr. Schoenfeld:

Since your column lately has contained many letters regarding trichomonas and yeast infections and the dread "non-specific vaginitis," here is my theory for whatever it's worth.

I had something or other of this sort on and off for eight years. But I haven't had a symptom for about a year. This is without any medication or change in habits and I am still on the pill as I have been for six years.

The difference? My present lover has blood type O-negative (I am O-positive). Previous periods of worse suffering involved two men, both type A. Since antigens and antibodies do appear in semen, saliva and vaginal fluid (I mean the anti-factors associated with ABO blood types), maybe blood type is a factor in those infamous itches.

Wonder if anyone else has noticed anything like this?

ANSWER: Some infertility problems in females have been traced to antibody reactions to the male's seminal fluid. So maybe you're on to something important, though one can't make conclusions from a sample of one.

Can we now expect to find blood typing reagents on milady's bedside table? Will love be vanquished by microscope slides and agglutination reactions? The answer to "What type of person do you like?" may be even more complicated than we know.

VD

Lower Abdominal Pain

Dear Dr. Schoenfeld:

I recently had intercourse with a guy I just met who has just left for Cal and I have no way of contacting him.

Well I've just begun to have pains when pressure is applied to the general area of the ovaries. I've never had these pains before and was just wondering if it's anything I should be concerned with.

Also, I think I might have certain psychological problems and would be interested in discussing them with a competent psychiatrist. But shit, who's got the bread: What do you suggest I do?

ANSWER: The pain you describe could be caused by a number of things including gonorrhea of the internal female organs.

Gonorrhea in the female often goes unnoticed at first, but any unusual vaginal discharge, burning on urination, itching or suspicion of contact with gonorrhea is sufficient reason for an examination by a physician.

Males usually know they have gonorrhea because of the discharge and painful urination. Females usually don't recognize the early symptoms. Every male who knows he has gonorrhea should notify all his female sexual contacts. Failure to do so may cause them to become sterile.

Information about free or low-cost psychotherapy should be available through your local public health department or nearest medical school.

Inadequate Diagnosis?

Dear Dr. Schoenfeld:

Three months ago I went to the hospital with a terrific pain in my side and a discharge. I thought I might have had the clap but the doctor said that I only had a bacterial disease in my sex organs and prescribed a suppository.

I still have the bothersome discharge and I experience great pain when I have a sexual contact. What is wrong?

P.S. Don't tell me to give up sex.

ANSWER: A pelvic examination for the symptoms you describe should include microscopic and bacterial culture examinations. Gonorrhea often involves a woman's uterus, Fallopian tubes and ovaries, causing lower abdominal pain and/or pain during intercourse. Inflammation and scarring of these organs may cause permanent sterility if the disease is not treated with penicillin or alternate antibiotics.

Don't delay seeing a gynecologist or the free Venereal Disease Clinic of your local health department.

A Teeny Hazard

Dear Dr. Schoenfeld:

My old man caught clap from some teeny-bopper chick. He is now taking medication.

Naturally we aren't balling right now. But can I catch it from simply sleeping with him?

Also, what kind of sexual activity can we safely engage in?

ANSWER: Gonorrhea is rarely transmitted except by direct sexual contact. The discharge of pus, of course, is infectious and must be avoided.

As for the kind of sexual activity you can safely engage in—you can think about what you'll do when your friend's physician tells him his infection has cleared up.

Good Friends

Dear Dr. Schoenfeld:

About one month ago, I had intercourse with a close friend who was visiting us from out of town. Since then I've had a lot of problems and have seen a gynecologist who says I have gonorrhea. I'm taking penicillin now and it's slowly clearing up.

My problem is I expect to see this guy soon and I know he's the only possible source of my infection. What should I say to him? Should I refuse any intercourse with him and tell him why? I don't want to lose his friendship.

ANSWER: If you're still being treated for gonorrhea you should not have intercourse—otherwise you'll return to him what he apparently gave you. Perhaps you should tell him what happened while emphasizing you regard gonorrhea as a disease and not a moral stigma. Had your friend felt the same way he could have saved you a lot of trouble.

Pelvic Inflammatory Disease

Dear Dr. Schoenfeld:

Because of two illegal abortions each followed by a serious infection, I have had a tendency toward infection of the tubes and ovaries. Six months ago my amorous activities got me in trouble again, this time gonorrhea.

The infection was undetected and improperly diagnosed until four months ago when I was doubled over with pain. Since then I have been to several clinics and several private doctors. Penicillin had good immediate results for the pain and fever phase, but the doctor who administered penicillin to me limited it to two shots and a pill prescription; then wanted me to take no more antibiotics, hoping my body could finish the job. This appealed to me because I've recently become interested in nutrition and the books I've been reading say protein and Vitamin C in large quantities fight infection.

Slowly, oh so slowly, I improved, with occasional pain, but feeling stronger overall. Then my doctor told me I could try intercourse in moderation. Two days after intercourse there was pain again, everywhere. My whole torso aches. The same thing when I smoke marijuana, or even exert myself in any way, like running on the beach, or mowing the lawn.

I went for follow-up tests to the Free Clinic last night because I can no longer afford my private doctor, not having worked since the great pain I experienced four months ago. The clinic doctor doubted that either test would prove positive after I explained the history of the case to him. The infection is too high up to be detected. He told me there might be pus trapped in my ovaries. He reiterated what I have already known and have been trying to adjust to—that I am likely sterile.

But now I am alarmed about even my own survival. It doesn't go away! It simply lies dormant awhile. When I try to cheer up what has become a very depressed disposition, it comes back, flares up, or whatever it is that it does. The doctor at the clinic admitted that he wasn't sure the treatment would effect a cure. He said it sometimes works.

I'm really beginning to think it's a matter of life and death, because I know it is impossible for me to lead a life like in a convent or rest home. I know *it's a matter of sanity because emotionally I'm used up. What do you suggest?*

ANSWER: Males who contract gonorrhea usually have burning and itching when urinating and a discharge of pus from the penis. But females may not notice any symptoms until the disease involves the uterus, ovaries and Fallopian tubes. Infection of these organs is called pelvic inflammatory disease (P.I.D.), the chief cause of which is gonorrhea. You've given a classic description of undiagnosed gonorrhea become chronic P.I.D.

P.I.D. is an important cause of sterility in females. Formerly found mainly in deprived socioeconomic groups, the disease is now frequently seen in college-age women. *Prevention of P.I.D. depends upon males* immediately notifying their sexual contacts whenever they know or suspect they have gonorrhea. Chronic P.I.D. often requires surgery for definitive treatment. If the clinic doctor refers you to a surgeon or gynecologist, follow his advice.

Proper nutrition is certainly important for good health, but I don't know of any diet or combination of foods that will cure gonorrhea. Penicillin is still effective in most cases of venereal disease. Although some people develop allergies to penicillin, the drug itself is relatively nontoxic. You could receive a shot daily for ten days or thirty days and chances are you'd suffer only from a sore bottom.

Strangely enough, many people are still unaware that local health departments operate free clinics for the diagnosis and treatment of VD.

Dear Dr. Schoenfeld:

Re: the girl with pelvic inflammatory disease caused by gonorrhea. I wonder if you would refer her to Jethro Kloos' book Back to Eden, *in particular p. 429, for herbal and water treatment of the infection. It's certainly worth a try. There* are *alternatives.*

ANSWER: Unless someone shows me some proof for these statements, beyond their appearing in print—I'm sticking to penicillin and other antibiotics.

I do believe other alternatives are possible but they haven't been discovered yet.

Inadequate Treatment

Dear Dr. Schoenfeld:

This past summer I enjoyed a fairly active sex life with several different men. However, somewhere along the line I managed to contract gonorrhea.

Around June or July I developed vaginal itching, but no discharge, and thought it was either a fungus or trichomonas infection which I've had before. I called my gynecologist and he gave me a prescription for vaginitis by telephone.

About a month later one of my boyfriends called me and said that he had a discharge from his penis and suspected that it was gonorrhea. He had worked in a V.D. clinic for a while and knew what the symptoms were. He had some tetracycline and took it for about five days.

I went to my doctor and got two shots of penicillin. O.K., so we're both clean—right? Neither of us had other contacts during the next month.

Then I saw another boyfriend (call him boyfriend #2). The next day I developed a violent itching. Again no discharge. A few days later boyfriend #2 called and said he had developed a discharge, had a smear taken and a positive diagnosis for gonorrhea was made. He said that up until he saw me, he had had no symptoms nor any other contacts.

I'm well aware that people are not always reliable about their sexual antics but I have good reason to believe both these men were telling me the truth about their sex life. As a result of all this I'm becoming extremely paranoid about sex. I can't have such a worry messing up my head and still enjoy my loving.

My questions are:

1) *Is it possible for a male to be a carrier of gonorrhea and have no symptoms?*
2) *Is it possible for me to be harboring the bug even after the treatment I had?*

ANSWER: Males most often are painfully aware of gonorrhea, but *some* may have no symptoms or symptoms so minor they are ignored. Gonorrhea and other venereal diseases have become so prevalent one can't afford not to see a physician if anything unusual is noticed about the genitals. Some studies have shown up to 20 percent of males have no symptoms.

Don't expect your doctor to make a diagnosis by telephone. The symptoms of trichomonas, fungus infections and gonorrhea may feel the same to the patient. While relatively few males are unaware of gonorrhea symptoms, most females contract the disease without knowing it.

Gonorrhea is becoming increasingly resistant to treatment with penicillin. Doses which were adequate a few years ago may now be too small. Some cases of gonorrhea are completely resistant to penicillin, necessitating use of other antibiotics. Laboratory examinations should be performed before and after treatment to insure eradication of the disease.

Of all the people mentioned in your letter, only boyfriend #2 was party to adequate medical care.

Oral Sex and VD

Dear Dr. Schoenfeld:

Would you please discuss in your column the possibility of contracting VD by oral-genital contact—cunnilingus or fellatio? What are the symptoms?

Can a sore throat indicate oral VD? I had a slightly sore throat (not painful) for several days and am uncertain if this was the sign of a slight cold (or flu) or the fact that I had oral-genital contact a week or so previously. I had no other symptoms.

ANSWER: Gonorrhea is usually transmitted through vaginal or anal intercourse. Gonorrhea of the mouth does occur but it's rarely diagnosed. The symptoms include a reddened sore throat.

The first stage of syphilis is a chancre or small, usually painless sore appearing anywhere sexual contact has been made. If a chancre is on the penis or vulva, oral-genital contact could transmit syphilis, a possibility well confirmed by medical experience.

The Pap Test

Dear Dr. Schoenfeld:

Last week I had a Pap test and I am having difficulty discovering what the results mean. The test came back with a 2+ (I understand 4+ to be a suspicion of cancer) and a recommendation for another Pap test in 3 months. It seems the cervix is inflamed. This is all I have been told. I am quite worried because I do not understand any of this.

a) *Why would they want me to have another Pap test if there is not some suspicion of cancer?*
b) *What is an inflamed cervix?*
c) *Do people who get a 2+ on one Pap smear tend to get a 3+ the next time? Is 2+ dangerous?*
d) *Do people with an inflamed cervix tend to get cancer?*
e) *What else can an inflamed cervix lead to?*

Last year I had erosion of the cervix; the doctor cauterized it. What is erosion? Why was it cauterized? What is cauterizing?

I am sorry to have so many questions but I have been totally unable to find a doctor willing to spend enough time to discuss my problem.

ANSWER: The Pap test is a simple, inexpensive method of detecting cancer of the cervix before the earliest symptoms, such as bleeding or an abnormal discharge, become apparent. Using a cotton swab or wooden spatula, the examining physician takes a smear sample from the cervix for microscopic examination of shed cells. Cancer produces cell changes identifiable to specially trained technicians. When the Pap smear is definitely suspicious of cancer the physician will take specimens of cervical tissue (a biopsy) for a more precise microscopic examination.

Improved detection and treatment methods have cut the death rate from uterine cancer in half during the last 30 years, but this malignancy still accounts for one-third the female cancer deaths. Most cancers of the uterus arise in the cervix or mouth of the womb and an estimated 9400 American women die from cervical cancer each year, according to The American Cancer Society. *Yet cancer of the cervix is 100 percent curable if detected in its early stages.* That's why Pap smears should be done at least once a year.

Inflammation, erosion, or infection of the cervix may be caused by a variety of conditions including yeast vaginitis and chronic irritation. These conditions often cause a false Pap test result—that's why your doctor wishes you to have another test after the inflammation has subsided.

Cervical cancer does seem to be related to irritation of the cervix. The disease is almost unknown, for example, in nuns or other groups of women who have never had sexual intercourse.

Wives of men whose religion dictates routine circumcision also have a very low rate of cervical cancer. Removal of the foreskin prevents accumulation of smegma, the cheesy substance thought to be the cancer-producing agent. Further evidence that good personal hygiene prevents this form of cancer comes from studies of American Indians. Cancer of the cervix is rare among Navajo Indians, a tribe known for exceptionally high standards of personal cleanliness. But American Indian women in general have a high rate of cervical cancer, as do other ethnic groups who live in poverty.

Inflammation of the cervix is often treated by cauterization, an ancient yet still valuable medical treatment. Heat, applied through an electric cautery, destroys the diseased tissue and the body's natural restorative powers can then complete the healing process. Cauterization of the cervix is painless. The cervix produces pain only when it is dilated, as in childbirth.

The Pap test was named for its developer, pathologist George Papanicolaou, M.D. I was a senior student at the University of Miami School of Medicine when Dr. Papanicolaou, then in his eighties, joined the faculty of our school. "Dr. Pap" died a few years ago, leaving as memorials the test bearing his name and the countless number of women whose lives he saved.

Vaginal Exercises

Dear Dr. Schoenfeld:

Everyone says that the penis size doesn't determine good sex; for me it's an important factor. I had a child 4 years ago but don't think I'm markedly bigger inside, at least my doctor says no.

I've always wished my husband were a little larger. (I love him dearly and have not had any extramarital affairs.) Since he can't expand, is there a way I can contract? Silicone injections? Douching with some mysterious chemical? Does any company make some device that I can insert before intercourse for a fuller feeling? Tell me.

My doctor just winks and smiles and says it's all in my head. That's not where I want it.

ANSWER: Have you been concerned about this for four years or just recently? At times, gynecologists perform a relatively easy surgical procedure which tightens a vagina unusually stretched by many deliveries. Before considering surgery though, try exercises for the muscles surrounding your vagina.

One exercise involves squeezing the same muscles used to prevent involuntary urination. Another is done by bearing down as if to expel stool from the bowel. These exercises should be done 20 times, three times a day. If the strength applied is gradually but consistently increased, results should be apparent within two weeks. It's not unusual for a woman to learn to flex independently the circular and longitudinal muscles encircling the vagina (the same muscles are used to control the anal and bladder sphincters). Pushing contracts one set of sphincter muscles while squeezing contracts the other set.

By placing a finger in the vagina or practicing on your husband, you (and he) will note the action of the two distinct muscle groups. Every woman (and her man) can benefit from increased vaginal muscle tone. The exercises are especially important following gynecological surgery or childbirth.

A San Francisco dancer told me she practices these exercises while doing her routine on stage. Other women practice several times a day while reading or working. Like the muscle-building exercises performed by weight lifters, the frequency and force used should be gradually increased. Okay, everyone out there—1, 2, 3 SQUEEZE!

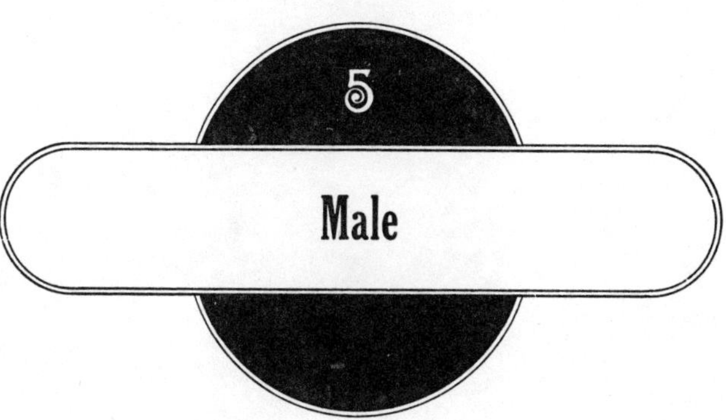

5

Male

Impotence

Dear Dr. Schoenfeld:

I have a sex problem that has really been giving me fits lately. Whenever I get in bed with a girl I do not stay hard long enough to have proper coitus. It's not that I don't get hard at all because I do easily—especially if the girl should give me manual stimulation.

In any case, by the time I begin intercourse I'm too soft. When I masturbate I have no trouble—so I think my potency is all right. Or is it? When I'm with a girl, I get an erection but it just doesn't last. I'm 22 and petting is a drag.

Isn't it more normal to stay hard until one is satisfied? Apparently my sex drive is weak. I doubt that it's psychological because sex doesn't hang me up—except for this problem.

What do you think?

ANSWER: Impotence is a very common sexual problem in older age groups but relatively rare in someone your age. Kinsey found that while less than 1 percent of males below the age of 35 suffered from permanent erectile impotence, by 70 years of age 27 percent of the men in his sample could no longer have sexual intercourse. But sexual potency may continue despite one's age—Kinsey's study included an 88-year-old man who continued to have sexual intercourse with his 90-year-old wife!

Masters and Johnson, the sex research team whose work has aided millions of people (including you, perhaps, if you'll read on), describe two types of impotency, primary and secondary. In primary impotency the male has never been able to "achieve and/or maintain an erection quality sufficient to accomplish successful coital connections." Masters and Johnson found causative factors in the men they treated included overbearing mothers, a suppressive religious background, self-depreciation and a tendency toward homosexuality.

Secondary impotence is diagnosed when a male cannot achieve coitus in 25 percent of his attempts. Occasional episodes of impotence occur in almost all men sometime in their lives, brought about by fatigue, recent sexual activity, overeating, psychological stress and certain drugs, most commonly alcohol, but including many tranquilizers. An episode of impotency caused by one of these factors shouldn't cause any alarm, but all too frequently a pattern is established. Fear of failure may so preoccupy a man he continues to fail—an illustration of not knowing there's "nothing to fear but fear itself."

Erectile problems following a bout with alcohol was the second most significant factor in Masters and Johnson's cases of secondary impotency. First in importance was a history of premature ejaculation, but it shouldn't be implied that most men who suffer from that problem will go on to become impotent (Masters and Johnson, incidentally, describe a technique so effective in treating premature ejaculation they believe it could be eliminated as a problem in our culture). Other factors causing secondary impotence were psychosocial influences, medications, injuries and diseases.

The first step in dealing with an impotency problem should be a thorough medical examination to rule out physical causes. Diabetes mellitus, for example, occasionally causes impotence. If a male is able to achieve an erection but not during intercourse an assumption can be made that the problem is not in his body.

Dr. Donald Hastings describes several types of psychological impotence in *Sexual Expression in Marriage* (Bantam Books). One is impotence of inexperience which he believes is common in young males, feelings of "ineptness, a fear of hurting the girl, an inability to reconcile the loved female with sexual passion, feelings of guilt and wrongdoing, fear of pregnancy" are all given as possible reasons. Philip Roth describes such an experience beginning on page 200 of *Portnoy's Complaint.*

I think you should consult your family physician—hopefully he'll have read the portions of Masters and Johnson's *Human Sexual Inadequacy* pertaining to your problem. You might also try calling the department of mental hygiene of your local health department to learn whether you're fortunate enough to live in one of the few cities in the United States offering clinics qualified to treat one of mankind's oldest problems.

See Your Physician

Dear Dr. Schoenfeld:

For the past six weeks or so I have been finding it extremely difficult to get a hard-on. I have also noticed that one of the testicles is becoming larger and the regular size one appears and feels like it has a growth coming on it. Do you think this would have anything to do with the erection problem?

Otherwise everything appears to be normal. Since I have always led a full sex life I would like to know what you think or if it would be advisable to see a doctor.

ANSWER: You should see a physician right away—either your own or a urologist. Referrals can be made through nearby medical schools or county medical societies.

Many people put off a visit to the doctor, even when they know something is wrong, for fear of confirming their worst suspicions. Paradoxical, true, but delaying medical treatment for this reason is a very common and sometimes very tragic occurrence.

An Elder's Advice

Dr. Hip,

I may be able to be of some help to your 22-year-old who suffered collapse during intercourse and to his partner or partners. It happens to all of us at some time if we live long enough. (I'll boast that it was some 40 years later for me.) When it happened to me it meant the end of games with coy or reluctant or only mildly interested women. It is only an affectionate woman who loves the sport and shows it and who promptly goes for her own touchdowns that kills that sinking feeling and brings out the best in me, and when that happens it's better than it ever was.

Masturbation

Dear Dr. Schoenfeld:
Could you explain how masturbation is done in males?

ANSWER: Read *Portnoy's Complaint.* Philip Roth's masterpiece is also destined for use as a text in helping psychotherapists understand the Jewish Mother Syndrome.

Blood After Masturbation

Dear Dr. Schoenfeld:
This morning when I masturbated my boyfriend, blood came out with the semen when he had his orgasm. He has no urinary problem, at least no burning sensation when he urinates and no blood shows at that time. As far as we know this is the first and only time this has happened. I'm concerned that the blood comes from the prostate or testicle and could indicate serious damage. As I can't make him go to see a doctor or urologist, I was hoping a letter to you might help. If you could spell out the possibilities for us, he could decide whether or not to see a doctor right away or wait to see if it happens again.

ANSWER: It's likely you only ruptured some capillaries within the penis through excessive zeal. There's probably nothing wrong now but the *only way to be certain* is for him to consult a physician.

Venereal Warts

Dear Dr. Schoenfeld:

I am a serviceman in Southeast Asia and my wife thinks I am having sexual relations here. Not so. But after arriving I noticed some pimple-like protrusions in my pubic area. I went to my sick bay where the corpsmen laughed them off as venereal warts!

This worried me so I wrote to my wife who is a Registered Nurse. She gave me rather a long medical term and said they were caused by gonorrhea. Now she is going to sue for divorce. I have checked with a few other medical sources and they all say the warts are not caused by sexual contact.

I am rather puzzled by the whole thing and would like to find out who is right. It doesn't seem possible that the service and civilian doctors could be 180 degrees out of line in diagnosing this problem.

ANSWER: Condyloma acuminata are warty growths thought to be caused by a virus. Their common name, "venereal warts," tends to perpetuate the false belief that they are caused by venereal diseases such as gonorrhea.

Venereal warts are seen more frequently in women than men and may appear anywhere on the vulva or within the vagina. At first the warts are small elevated growths the size, perhaps, of a mole. Later they become quite large, giving a mulberrylike appearance. Conditions which seem to favor growth of venereal warts in females are a profuse vaginal discharge, obesity, infrequent bathing and pregnancy.

Treatment for venereal warts is similar in males and females. A solution is applied directly to the warts which causes them to shrink and disappear. Often one or more reapplications are necessary. Some mild discomfort may be noted in the surrounding area but the procedure is much less painful than you might imagine.

N.S.U. (Nonspecific Urethritis)

Dear Dr. Schoenfeld:

Recently I came down with nonspecific urethritis or NSU. My doctor told me that NSU was non-communicable yet he advised me not to have sexual intercourse for at least a week. This sounds self-contradictory to me. Is it?

If left untreated will NSU eventually clear up?

ANSWER: Nonspecific urethritis may cause the same initial symptoms in the male as gonorrhea—itching, burning and a discharge from the penis. But microscopic and bacteriologic examination of the discharge does not show the characteristic coffee-bean-shaped gonococcus bacteria which cause gonorrhea.

Since no one organism can be shown to cause the symptoms, this troublesome ailment is known as nonspecific urethritis (NSU). Treatment usually consists of a broad-spectrum antibiotic such as tetracycline. Often, the treatment and the drip continue on and on and on. Your physician advised against sexual intercourse to lessen the possibility of irritating already inflamed tissues.

The Cream did a song called "NSU" which consists, in part, of what seem to be wails of anguish.

VD

The Sound of One Hand

Dear Dr. Schoenfeld:

A friend of mine has been forbidden by his doctor to indulge in intercourse until a nasty bit of the clap is entirely cleared up. If any of his girlfriends should decide to employ digital manipulation to achieve orgasm would this result in a case of the "hand-clap"?

ANSWER: I applaud the concern you have for your friend and his friends. Most physicians believe all sexual activity should be avoided while treatment for gonorrhea is underway.

The symptoms of gonorrhea in the male are itching, burning and pain on urination and a discharge from the urethra.

Gay Men and VD

Dear Dr. Schoenfeld:

I have seen several columns of yours dealing with venereal diseases, but they dealt with the problems of straight guys and girls. Would you please inform the gay members of your reading audience that they too can contract V.D.? Not only via the genitals, but anally and orally as well?

Proctitis can be just as uncomfortable as pelvic inflammatory diseases (P.I.D.). Most doctors, private and public, will not be shocked by seeing a real live homosexual. There is no onus to an anus check.

Yin-Yang

Dear Dr. Schoenfeld:

Sometimes you hear that very tight clothing around the scrotum of the male can cause sterility. I just can't believe that. Athletes, particularly professionals, wear jock straps several hours daily, ballet dancers live day in and day out with tight leotards, and male fashions today may often call for very tight slim underwear. What is the truth about tight clothing and male sexuality? What does medical research show?

ANSWER: Writer Martin Schneider posed the same question in a different way. He asked, "What is the lethal factor formed by males' wearing uptight trousers?"

A brief discussion of the function of the scrotum is necessary in order to explain why "uptight" trousers and underwear are thought to have an effect on male fertility.

The reason seems to be that man's body temperature of 98.6° F or 37° C is too high for the production of sperm. During the development of the male fetus, the testes normally descend from his body cavity into the scrotal sac. Males with two undescended testicles will be infertile unless corrective measures are taken before the age of five or six. The chief function of the scrotum seems to be to separate the testicles from the rest of the body in order to maintain them at a temperature optimal for the production of sperm.

Cold weather causes the cremaster muscles to contract, thus drawing the scrotum closer to the body (fear can stimulate the same protective reflex). The "cremasteric reflex" is one of the tests in a neurologic examination. To observe the effect of this test, scratch the inner side of your thigh (or that of a very close friend) with your fingertip. You should see the testicle withdraw on that side.

An article in the April 27, 1968, *Journal of the A.M.A.* reported the results of applying heat and cold to the scrotum. Authors Robinson, Rock and Menkin of the Rock Reproduction Clinic found that heating the scrotum depressed the production of sperm, while cooling the scrotum increased sperm production.

In normal subjects, exposure of the scrotum to a 150 watt electric light bulb for 30 minutes on 14 consecutive days caused a decrease in sperm production. But half the subjects in their experiments reported a considerable increase in libido two or three weeks after heating the scrotum. Application of an ice bag to the scrotum for 30 minutes a day on 14 consecutive days following the exposure to heat stimulated spermatogenesis so much that the mean sperm count was nearly three times the sperm count before treatment with either heat or cold. The authors postulated that this might be an effective treatment for those with low sperm counts, often a cause of male sterility.

The authors suggest that in normal males fertility could possibly be diminished by sitting on hot machinery, wearing tightly woven protective clothing or by taking long hot baths.

"Even relatively simple alterations in male dress, in deference to fashion, conceivably may render a healthy young man comparatively infertile."

They believe that actively cooling the testicles by swimming in cold water may serve as a physiological means of increasing fertility.

Sequential application of heat and cold is well known to lusty Scandinavians and others who steam in saunas before leaping naked into the snow or an icy pool (arrgh!).

What does a Scotsman wear under his kilt? Most likely a higher sperm count than found in men wearing close-fitting underwear and tight jeans. Togas anyone?

Referral

Dear Dr. Schoenfeld:

In a heavy petting session should a guy unzip himself and place his organ in his date's hand or wait for her to do this for him?

ANSWER: Write to Dear Abby.

6

Conception and Contraception

Misconceptions

"Unwanted pregnancies accounted for about 40 percent of births in the United States between 1960–68," said Charles Westoff, Ph.D., Princeton University office of population research.

Unwanted Miracle

Dear Dr. Schoenfeld:

Many years ago when I was a lad the family doctor advised me to get laid. When I protested that I didn't want to take a chance of getting a girl pregnant, he described a technique whereby both parties could have all the pleasure of intercourse with none of the risks.

His instructions were to have the girl clasp my penis between her thighs so tight that clitoral contact would be made and using Vaseline for a lubricant carry on as usual.

As far as I was concerned, the difference between internal and external sensation was trivial. Some girls found it sufficient, some not—but it was better than nothing and did not involve either loss of virginity or pregnancy.

ANSWER: You were lucky. Many cases of pregnancy have occurred in virgins as a result of techniques similar to the one you describe. If ejaculated semen reaches the vaginal entrance, miraculous results may follow.

Coitus Interruptus

Dear Dr. Schoenfeld:

William Baird, birth control expert, is quoted as saying:

"You'd be surprised how naive about sex some of those bright college kids are. Some of them believe they can prevent pregnancy by withdrawal."

Now, just what is wrong with "pulling out" as a means of contraception?

ANSWER: Coitus interruptus is a risky means of contraception—and a drag as well.

Small amounts of semen may be deposited in the vagina before the sensation of ejaculation occurs. Studies have shown this amount of fluid contains thousands of spermatozoa.

Upward Mobility

Dear Dr. Hip:

I know that I can get pregnant even without actually having intercourse if my boyfriend lies on top of me and we don't have any clothes on.

But what if one of us has underwear on and the other one doesn't?

ANSWER: Unless you're wearing a wet suit or some other impermeable garment you'd better lay off. Spermatozoa strain mightily to reach their goal.

More Body Education Needed

Dear Dr. Schoenfeld:

I've been told all the sperm is ejected after the first ejaculation. After that, the story goes, one may have another orgasm, or several, but for 36 hours or so, he won't be able to father a child.

If I could do it with a rubber at night and without it in the morning, I'd be happy.

ANSWER: I hope you read this soon. The amount of sperm does decrease with each subsequent orgasm during a fixed period of time but you can certainly impregnate your friend(s) each and every time. The average emission of semen may contain 500 million spermatozoa and each one could conceivably cause a girl to conceive.

Orgasms and Pregnancy

Dear Dr. Hip Pocrates:

A chick I know told me recently chicks can only get pregnant if they come at the same time as their dude. I was under the impression that there were many mothers who had never had an orgasm.

Does the female orgasm have any effect on pregnancy?

ANSWER: Your friend may find out she's wrong the hard way. Some physicians think orgasms late in pregnancy can cause premature labor but your friend's belief must have come from an old wife.

Sex and Menstruation

Dear Dr. Schoenfeld:

Are there any medical reasons for not having intercourse during menstruation?

ANSWER: There are no known medical reasons against having sexual intercourse during menstruation. In fact, some women feel more erotic at this time.

The Rhythm Method

Dear Dr. Schoenfeld:

A friend of mine informed me that it is possible to be pregnant even though I just had my period. Is this so? If so, is this a rare thing?

ANSWER: A woman with a 28-day cycle will normally ovulate on the fourteenth day, counting the first day of menstruation as day one. The optimum time for achieving pregnancy, given this cycle, is day 14, but wide variations are found from one female to another.

The "safest" times during a woman's menstrual cycle are five days before, during, and three days following menstruation. But pregnancy has been known to occur even when intercourse took place only during menstruation.

The rhythm method is notoriously poor as a method for birth control.

On Her Mind

Dear Dr. Schoenfeld:

I am 18 and have had sexual relations on and off since the age of 14. I find sex wonderful and beautiful. The boys (men) involved have been those I dated for more than 4 months steadily.

I'm Catholic and always vow to never sleep with anyone again, but somehow I always do. I mean like it's on my mind a lot.

I secretly fear that I am sterile and have used few precautions. A couple of times my lovers have, but last year we were having relations 3–4 times a week and I didn't become pregnant.

Do you think something is wrong with me? I tried going to a doctor to find out but I was 17 then and my mother wouldn't give me permission for a pelvic examination. Could it be that my lovers (5 in all) have all been sterile, that I am sterile or that we have all been extremely lucky?

ANSWER: Most gynecologists would not be concerned about possible infertility in a female until she had been with one man for a year or more using no contraceptive methods. But you should have a pelvic examination by your family physician or gynecologist now that you're old enough.

The chances are you've just been fortunate. Whatever else you press, don't press your luck.

Delayed Menstruation

Dear Dr. Schoenfeld:

I don't know whether I'm pregnant or whether my system is just very fouled up. The first time I ever had intercourse was two months ago. Ten days later I had my period but only a very little. I haven't had my period since.

Is it possible for me to be pregnant? I thought after having my period it was impossible but I'm now 17 days late and very worried. During the past few months I've been doing a lot of drugs—smoke, diet pills, downs, meth, MDA and psilocybin. I did the last 2 during the past weekend. Could these drugs be affecting my system causing me to be late? I really don't know what to think.

If I am pregnant, how do I go about getting an abortion? Do I have to tell my parents? It would just hurt them so much. I'm 19 (20 in February) and am going to school at the University of Miami; I have so much on my mind right now I'm having a hard time doing my school work. In fact, I'm having trouble doing everything. I never thought I'd have this problem. Even now I can hardly conceive the idea. I can't believe I'm writing you either.

ANSWER: Your menstrual period could be delayed by the drugs you mention, emotional upset (such as fear of pregnancy) or pregnancy. A pregnancy test obtained through a gynecologist or Planned Parenthood would answer your question very quickly.

If you should be pregnant Planned Parenthood also provides counseling services, including referrals for abortions when indicated.

Nonprescription Contraceptives

Douching and Contraception

Dear Dr. Hip Pocrates:

I was remembering the old trick of using a shaken up Coke as a douche in order not to get pregnant. Is there any truth to this?

ANSWER: Douching is a most unreliable way of preventing pregnancy. Birth control is not among the things that go better with Coke.

Vaginal Foam

Dear Dr. Schoenfeld:

My girlfriend and I rely on a vaginal foam to stifle the stork. I have noticed that after about a half hour of vigorous, uninterrupted intercourse, a large pile of foam appears on the bed.

The amount is so great that it worries me whether or not there can be enough left in the proper place to be effective. Are my worries justified or don't things work that way?

ANSWER: Even if you didn't work yourself up into a lather your chances of conceiving a child are increased if you use a vaginal foam rather than contraceptive pills or a diaphragm. Vaginal foams, however, are certainly more convenient and probably as effective as condoms. Vaginal foams, by the way, need not be inserted immediately before sexual intercourse ("the pause that depresses").

A former secretary spumed forth the information that she uses a double dose of foam for safety's sake.

Dear Dr. Schoenfeld:

Every now and then I meet a girl who uses Emko vaginal foam to prevent pregnancy. It seems to do the job alright (I think) but there is one thing which really is annoying—the taste! Why does Emko taste so bad? I've sampled one or two other brands and they're no better. What do you suggest?

ANSWER: Your complaint is quite common and I'm sure the Emko Company would be interested in your comments. Write to them at 7912 Manchester Avenue, St. Louis, Mo. 63143. "Give them a tongue-lashing." (Sec'y's note)

Dear Dr. Schoenfeld:

Since some chicks rely upon those vaginal foams, jellies, etc., when are the manufacturers of these products going to start producing them in flavors? Chocolate's my favorite.

ANSWER: Multiflavored vaginal douches are such a profitable venture they were reported in *Time*'s advertising section. Maybe contraceptive foam and jelly manufacturers will also respond to changing American tastes.

Dear Dr. Hip:

Could you please tell me the chances of getting pregnant on the first occasion of sexual intercourse? I am 13.

Also could you tell me some easy ways of birth control? Is the Pill a prescription thing? If it is, is there any other way I could not get pregnant?

I don't want to ask my mother these things because she thinks I am very clean. I have not had intercourse yet but if I do I would like to know these things.

ANSWER: You'd be surprised at the number of girls who become pregnant the first time they attempt sexual intercourse. (They were, too!)

Contraceptive vaginal foams, jellies and suppositories are available without prescription but they are not as effective as diaphragms, intrauterine loops or birth control pills. Planned Parenthood clinics offer classes in which these and other contraceptive methods are discussed in detail. Some PP clinics offer special classes for teenagers.

But I wonder if you're prepared in other ways. Maybe it was just a slip of the pen (maybe), but why do you think sex is dirty?

Well, Hip—

You've done it. Roused my utter disgust.

Recently a female child, 13 years old, appealed to you about sex—and what did you tell her? In effect, go ahead, just don't get pregnant, and "what makes you think sex is dirty?"

Sex isn't dirty (with qualifications) but venereal disease is—*a curse that affects even the yet unborn let alone the personal misery and ruin it can cause. Also, one contact, like pregnancy, is enough. Why didn't you warn her? And you are an M.D.? Aren't you obligated? God, help us.*

My heart goes out to that poor child, still innocent. Publish this, will you? She might read it and at least be warned. I am a mother and concerned.

Taking No Chances

Dear Dr. Schoenfeld:

If I use a condom and my chick uses a contraceptive vaginal foam when we are balling are the chances of conception much lower than if either of the two is used alone?

ANSWER: Yes, much lower.

Planned Parenthood

Dear Dr. Schoenfeld:

Could you please tell me how and where I can get a convenient contraceptive?

Unfortunately, it is impossible for me to get any by prescription as I am 17, single and living with my parents.

P.S. I hope that you understand "convenient" to mean something I would not have to use at an inopportune time. This can tend to be mood-breaking at best.

ANSWER: It's true that many private physicians are reluctant to prescribe birth control pills or other contraceptive devices for minor females without the consent of parents. But, fortunately, birth control advice and/or devices are available to females of ANY AGE at most Planned Parenthood centers. If, for some reason you don't want to go to the Planned Parenthood Center in your community, you can go to another one. They will help you regardless of where you live. The fees are set on a sliding scale depending on income and number of dependents, but "no one is ever turned away."

During the first visit to Planned Parenthood, a nurse will conduct a class in methods of contraception. Males are welcome. Next comes a short intake session with an interviewer. Following the brief interview, a physician gives a breast and pelvic examination, including a cancer or Pap smear. Contraceptive supplies are then issued.

Most girls choose contraceptive pills because they are 100 percent effective when used according to instructions. Some, however, prefer to use an intrauterine device (I.U.D., loop), diaphragm or vaginal foam. The rhythm method is taught also, even though it's most unreliable.

Planned Parenthood is a voluntary agency which provides many services besides birth control information and devices. They maintain an infertility referral service for couples unable to have children, premarital counseling, pregnancy testing, and a referral service to private physicians for medical problems, tubal ligations and vasectomies. They also conduct educational programs for community groups and information and training for professional workers in medicine, social work, religion, social science and public health. Some PP centers maintain abortion clinics.

Fifty years ago, Margaret Sanger and her sister, nurse Ethel Byrne, were arrested and imprisoned in New York City for the "crime" of dispensing information about birth control. Similar arrests continued until recently when the Supreme Court decreed that laws forbidding the prescribing of birth control devices by physicians were unconstitutional.

A related question was the right of a physician to perform an abortion when requested to do so by a woman. This battle was won in 1973 through a historic U.S. Supreme Court decision stating that abortions were the concern of women and their physicians, not the state.

The Pill

Dear Dr. Schoenfeld:

Recent stories about the dangers of the "pill" have made me really scared. Some of my friends have stopped taking them and I'm ready to do the same. What do you think?

ANSWER: My bias is that of a pleasure-loving male, but here's what I think of the situation:

Birth control pills, when taken as directed, are the best means known to prevent conception—short of abstinence. Many women experience unpleasant symptoms, especially when they first begin using the "pill"; these may include nausea, vomiting, headaches, nervousness, depression, breakthrough bleeding, spotting, breast enlargement and/or tenderness, and weight gain. In short, a simulation of early pregnancy symptoms. Other women have none of these effects.

Of greater concern are the reports of blood clots (some leading to death) and the possibility of inducing cancer. An English study reported that women using birth control pills had seven to ten times the rate of death and illness caused by blood clots when compared to non-"pill"-using females. The statistical breakdown looked like this:

"Pill" users between 20 and 34 had a mortality rate from blood clots of 1.5 per 100,000, while non-"pill"-users in the same age group had a mortality rate of 0.2 per 100,000. "Pill" users between 35 and 44 had a mortality rate of 3.9 per 100,000, while non-"pill"-users in the same bracket had a rate of 0.5 per 100,000. "Pill" users between 20 and 44 had a hospitalization rate for illness caused by blood clots of 47 per 100,000, while the figure for non-"pill"-users was 5 per 100,000.

In other words, women are not dropping like flies due to birth control pills, but they do have statistically significant increased mortality and morbidity rates in England compared with non-users. We don't yet know whether the new low-dose pills lower the incidence of blood clots. What about the possibility of contraceptive pills causing cancer? No case of cancer has ever been attributed to the "pill" during the ten years they have been extensively used. Nonetheless, since estrogens are known to stimulate certain cancers, yearly or semiannual gynecologic examinations, including Pap smears, should be performed on all women using contraceptive pills. In fact, every woman should have an annual pelvic exam. The results of using the "pill" for 20 or 30 years, or the effect on succeeding generations, are unknown.

Every woman, then, must decide for herself whether she wishes to use the "pill," with its *almost* certain contraceptive properties (nothing is certain) and slight but real risks of illness and death. The dangers of pregnancy remain greater than the dangers to users of contraceptive pills. Birth control pills should not be taken by women with a history of thrombophlebitis, strokes, impaired liver function or cancer.

Panic resulting from sensational news stories a few years ago caused an upsurge in unwanted pregnancies and many abortions, legal and illegal. Congress is hardly an appropriate place to evaluate a drug.

Pills from Mom

Dear Dr. Schoenfeld:

I am in my late 40's, a mother of 3 children and I would like to ask you about birth control pills for my daughter. She is 16—excuse me, in two months she will be 17—and has been going steady for over a year. At this age could the pills be harmful?

Remembering back to when I was a teenager I know how it was to neck and become emotional with a boy. Do you or would you advise my obtaining birth control pills for her? She is a very bright girl with an open mind—but coming from her mother do you think she would resent it?

She is a little difficult to communicate with where things like sex, etc., are concerned. She gets embarrassed and I'm not sure whether it is because I am not able to discuss it properly with her or whether she feels she knows enough.

ANSWER: I discussed your letter with a freckle-faced member of my research staff just a few years older than your daughter. She suggests telling her you think a girl her age should know all about birth control even if she's not having sex.

Parents and children often find these matters embarrassing, even in the most enlightened families, so a visit to your family doctor or a physician she chooses would be helpful. If you live in an area served by Planned Parenthood your daughter could attend one of their classes on birth control methods. Some Planned Parenthood clinics conduct classes especially for teenagers. Birth control pills are prescribed for girls of 16 and younger but it's best not to use them until growth has stopped.

And for those girls who didn't have so concerned a mother there's a book called *Single and Pregnant* by Ruth I. Pierce, published by Beacon Press ($5.95). *Single and Pregnant* answers such questions as "What do I do?", "Where do I go?" and "What do I need?" Being single and pregnant isn't so scandalous or difficult today as it was just a few years ago, but for most girls it's still a giant hassle, best avoided by sound sex education and preventive measures.

Dear Dr. Schoenfeld:

I would like to congratulate the mother who wanted her daughter to take birth control pills. When I was 17 I had been going with a guy for a year and a half and both my parents asked us (my boyfriend and I) if I wanted to take the pill. My mother is a nurse and my father a doctor.

The four of us discussed it, its effects on me and on our

relationship. My boyfriend and I decided we didn't need it then and thanked them. Since then I've loved and respected my parents so much more. I'm now 19, a freshman in college and my boyfriend is 22. We are still in love and using the "pill." When we felt it was time for us to use birth control methods we went to my parents.

A Daughter In Love—with her parents and her fellow.

How Long Is Safe?

Dear Dr. Schoenfeld:

My physician accepts the theory that one should go off birth control pills every 4 years in order to prevent future difficulties in pregnancy.

Since I hope to have my first baby in around 2 years, but don't want to go off contraceptive pills, I'd like to know what evidence supports this theory.

ANSWER: Because birth control pills have been used clinically only for the past ten years or so, many physicians take their patients off the pills at periodic intervals as a precautionary measure. Time limits on the use of birth control pills had been recommended by manufacturers and the U.S. Food and Drug Administration but when no adverse effects from long term use of "the pill" were discovered these recommendations were abandoned.

A Reliable Contraceptive?

Dear Dr. Schoenfeld:

Is there any danger of a girl getting pregnant during her period while she's on the pill?

My girlfriend started taking birth control pills but there are only 20 pills in each pack leaving 8 days per month (including her period) "unprotected." Since you wrote that it is possible (though improbable) for a girl to get pregnant during her period, does a 20 day pill supply give true 28 day protection?

Further, she tells me that the pills are rather small. Would they still be effective if one were to get caught in her mouth and dissolve there, rather than in her stomach?

P.S. Please answer in the next two weeks.

ANSWER: Birth control pills act by preventing ovulation, the release of eggs from the ovaries. Spermatozoa may find their way to the customary trysting place, the Fallopian tubes, but won't find there the objects of their affection.

Hormones contained in birth control pills also nurture blood vessels and the tissue lining within the uterus. Withdrawal of these hormones at the end of a 20- (or 21-) day pill cycle causes the uterine wall lining to degenerate and slough. The result is similar to normal menstrual bleeding.

Many medications are effective when dissolved and absorbed by mucous membranes such as those lining the mouth, vagina and rectum. Birth control pills should be swallowed whole. But if they are dissolved in the mouth they'll either be absorbed in the mouth or swallowed.

Birth control pills give full protection throughout the menstrual cycle. So far as we know, the only girls to become pregnant while on the pill are those who can't count.

A Strange Tale

Dear Dr. Schoenfeld:

I have a story I would like to relate to you. Here it is:

Herb visited Linda in December and again in July. He did not see her in the six months in between and therefore did not ball her during that time.

Linda stopped taking her birth control pills early in April and became pregnant later that month. She claims that Herb is the father. That she carried around the sperm (or the fertilized egg) from December until April and when she stopped taking birth control pills became pregnant. She is now four months pregnant.

A psychiatrist told Herb that this is possible. I personally don't believe it. Have you ever heard of this? Do you think it could happen?

ANSWER: Linda will have to accept some other explanation. Pregnancy could occur, for example, without intercourse if the sperm were deposited at or near the vaginal entrance. Perhaps Herb misinterpreted the psychiatrist's words. He might have said something like, "Well . . . anything is possible, but . . ."

Spermatozoa rarely remain alive in the vagina more than 2 or 3 days whether or not a woman is taking birth control pills. Deep freezing can maintain sperm cells in a state of suspended animation for long periods of time. But your friend would have had to be quite literally frigid for this phenomenon to occur.

Forgetting to Take a Pill

Dear Dr. Hip:

My husband and I are disagreeing about something and we hope you can solve it. A lot of my friends have this problem, too.

What happens if you forget to take your birth control pill? How many pills can you not take without trouble? My husband says you can forget 4 a month with no problem. But my sister-in-law usually forgot to take about 4 a month and now she's pregnant.

ANSWER: If you should miss taking a birth control pill, take two the next day. If something is working on your head and you've forgotten two, three or four days in a row, take the missed pills when you do remember. Use an additional method of contraception during the remainder of that cycle.

The chance of conception occurring when one pill is missed is small if you "double up" the following day. But the risk increases with each missed pill. Any woman who forgets her birth control pills four days in a row or four times in a cycle probably has an unconscious wish to become pregnant. Other means of contraception should be used until she clearly knows what she wants to do.

Vending the Pill

Birth control pills can be purchased from a vending machine at the University of the Philippines, according to the *Philippine Collegian.* The machine carries several popular brands of "the pill" and was installed by the school's student council to reduce the number of unwanted pregnancies.

We don't handle "the pill" so casually, and with good reason, but relatively few American student health services provide birth control information and devices, though many are entirely supported by student fees. It's strange that students at these schools have not insisted upon provision of contraceptive devices.

Pill Putdown

Dear Dr. Hip Pocrates:

I'm putting down "the pill." Now my body can return to its natural cycle and suddenly I'm free.

Sure this means I can't ball everyone—nor contract so many bloody diseases. If I get pregnant maybe that is what's supposed to happen. What were women made for?

Plus no more hang-ups! It's really a drag not to be able to make love because you don't have your pill with you—situation comedies. Or having to go clear across town to get it or where am I going to get them this month.

Look at it this way. If you have to carry your pills around, then you have to carry a purse—so you fill it up with cigarettes, cosmetics, money, all life's hang-ups. And you have to tote it around with you wherever you go. That's no freedom, that's a burden.

I'd much rather just let my body do what it wants to do.

ANSWER: Birth control pills are the most reliable means of contraception, but they're not advisable for every female. Perhaps the contraceptive device best suited for you would be an intrauterine device (I.U.D., "loop").

The "Morning After" Pill

Doc:

The other night this cat and I balled. I'm not on the pill or anything and like we went all the way, man. It was really beautiful.

What I want to know is, is there anything I can do before my period starts (in 3 weeks) to make *sure it* starts? *Should I go to the doctor's or what? Like man, let me know soon before it's too late. Cause my old man and I* can't *hack a child yet!*

ANSWER: The "morning after" pill presently in use is actually an old drug used for a new purpose. When *diethylstilbestrol* is given in sufficient quantity over a four or five day period it prevents pregnancy *if taken within three days after intercourse.* Some nausea and vomiting is common but most girls put up with this minor discomfort rather than risk an unwanted pregnancy.

You should use diethylstilbestrol as a "morning after" pill only if you absolutely do not want the child. Should it fail to work you must obtain an abortion because daughters born to women given diethylstilbestrol during pregnancy often develop cancer of the vagina.

But like man, it's easier to prevent pregnancy with birth control pills, intrauterine devices (I.U.D. s, loops,) diaphragms, condoms, or spermicidal foams and jellies (in decreasing order of effectiveness).

Intrauterine Devices

Dear Dr. Schoenfeld:

Why are doctors reluctant to prescribe an I.U.D. (intrauterine device) for a woman who has not had any children?

ANSWER: Nulliparous women have more bleeding and cramping and expel I.U.D.s more frequently than those who have borne children. Newer I.U.D. models, though, have allowed their use by many females who haven't had children.

I.U.D.s work well for most women after the initial discomfort of insertion and increased bleeding and cramping which follow in the next month or so. Some women aren't uncomfortable at any time because of their I.U.D.s.

But others have suffered severe pain, a uterus pierced by the I.U.D., severe pelvic infections or pregnancy due to a dislodged loop. And more than one baby has entered this world clutching an I.U.D. in his hand, perhaps with glee.

Unfortunately, we do not yet have a method of birth control both safe and effective.

Tubal Ligation

Dear Dr. Schoenfeld:

If a married girl (age 19) wants a tubal ligation must she first have had at least one child? Or can she only obtain this operation because of infection or some other medical reason?

Is it possible to have a spinal anesthetic? How long must a person be hospitalized? And finally, what is the approximate cost?

ANSWER: Tubal ligations involve cutting the Fallopian tubes (the passages between the ovaries and the uterus) and tying off the severed ends. The result is usually permanent sterilization: reconnecting the Fallopian tubes after such a procedure rarely results in a successful pregnancy.

Total hospitalization for a standard tubal ligation is about four days and the cost runs between $600 and $800. When the surgery is done following delivery of a baby the cost is less and only an extra day's stay in the hospital is necessary. Spinal anesthesia may be used.

But I doubt if a reputable physician would do a tubal ligation on a 19-year-old girl who had never borne a child. You have left about 20 potential childbearing years. Once a tubal ligation is performed it's too late to change your mind.

Dear Dr. Schoenfeld:

About tubal ligations: May I submit an enthused testimonial for tubal ligations by a new method using a laparoscope (a telescopelike device).

The only incisions were an invisible one in my navel and a tiny pinpoint scar a few inches away, on my abdomen—two band-aids when I awoke.

The surgeon fills the belly cavity with carbon dioxide gas, distending it and very easily locating the Fallopian tubes and uterus visibly with a flexible light and "scope." Then through the pinhole opening he cuts and cauterizes the tubes. A few stitches repair everything—they fall out a week later.

I experienced no discomfort at all afterwards—I swear that I could have walked home as soon as I woke up from the anesthesia (Demerol, curare, sodium pentothal). They keep one overnight for observation, mostly because it is traditional, I understand. The operation itself took 20 minutes. Because I am a welfare mother, the state paid for it.

Since the doctors, staff and even the food were so good, the only complaint I have is that one does have to get shaved and await one's pubic hair getting long and soft again. Boo!

Five days after the operation I made one follow-up visit to the GYN outpatient clinic, gave my groovy doctor a bottle of wine and that was it! He just told me to remember to get a Pap smear once a year, and good-bye.

The welfare even paid for the sitter, for the time I was hospitalized. I am 29, with two super kids and in the initial interview I didn't have to lie or threaten Women's Lib, or anything. The going attitude in this clinic is that if a woman is grown-up and rational and seems to know what she wants, they will help her to control her fertility (also they saw my two-year-old kicking up his heels—maybe that helped!).

Love, and hooray for stopping the baby machine when that's what fits one's life.

Vasectomies

Dear Dr. Schoenfeld:

I've been married for five years now. A little over seven years ago, my husband, he was 18 then, had a vasectomy (clip job, he calls it) in order to make him sterile.

He has been sorry that he did it but what was done was done. We decided we would adopt a couple of children next year or the year after.

But believe it or not, I am pregnant. Missed last March

but didn't worry. Finally my doctor insisted on a test at the end of May and that proved it.

My husband won't believe that he is the father. I have no reason to lie to you—I don't know you nor you me. Another man hasn't touched me in 6 years. My doctor told him it was possible for the vasectomy to heal and asked to examine him but he thinks my M.D. would lie (I think maybe he suspects my doctor).

Now he has said that he does not blame me for wanting a child but insists on knowing who this "mythical" man is.

It would make him the happiest man on earth if he just knew it was his baby.

ANSWER: A vasectomy is a simple surgical procedure often performed in a physician's office. Two small openings are made in the scrotum in order to cut and tie off both vasa deferentia, the spaghetti-like tubes which transport sperm from the testicles. Vasectomies ALMOST always cause permanent sterility. Since attempts to reunite the severed ends of the vas deferens are usually unsuccessful, few physicians would perform a vasectomy on an 18-year-old.

Rarely, the severed ends reunite spontaneously and this apparently has happened in your husband's case. Any family physician or urologist could examine your husband's semen microscopically and tell him whether he could father a child.

The Perfect Contraceptive

Another method of preventing unwanted pregnancies was proposed recently by India's Family Planning Minister, Sripati Chandrasekhar.

The cheapest and safest method of family planning, he said, was abstinence. Abstinence for a year would be of great benefit for the individual and the country, the Family Planning Minister said in a speech at Poona University. Sure.

Conception

Signs of Pregnancy

Dear Dr. Hip Pocrates:

I had intercourse for the first time last night (I'm 17 years old). I have heard that it's supposed to be painful the first time, but it didn't hurt and I didn't bleed.

What I am wondering about is whether there are any signs that would show I'm pregnant (morning sickness, etc.)?

Could you please answer this soon? I'm very frightened.

ANSWER: The first sign of pregnancy is usually a missed menstrual period. Other early signs are a feeling of fullness and enlargement of the breasts, darkening of the nipples, and nausea and vomiting, especially in the morning.

Laboratory tests for pregnancy can now be done in a matter of minutes. A sample of urine or blood is taken 10 to 14 days after the missed period.

Many girls experience no pain or bleeding when they first have intercourse. But an unwanted pregnancy can cause you needless suffering. You'd better see your family physician, a gynecologist or the nearest Planned Parenthood Clinic soon to learn about contraceptive measures.

Fertility Problem

Dear Dr. Schoenfeld:

Everyone writes about preventing conception; but we never see anything about how to get pregnant. I am married and we've been trying for almost a year.

Do you have any tips on how to make conception more likely?

ANSWER: Most physicians consider a couple to have an infertility problem if pregnancy does not occur after a year of normal marital relations without the use of contraceptives. But, as you point out, little information is given about increasing the chances of conception.

Assuming a 28-day menstrual cycle (the first day of bleeding is day one), the most fertile period is on or about the fourteenth day. You can buy a highly calibrated thermometer at your pharmacy which will help you determine just when ovulation occurs. The female's body temperature usually drops one or one and a half days before ovulation. One or two days after ovulation there is a temperature rise of about 0.7 degrees Fahrenheit and this temperature increase continues through the rest of the menstrual cycle. The fertile period ends three days after the rise in temperature.

Four or five days of abstinence will increase the volume of semen. Following sexual intercourse in the "missionary" or male superior position, the woman's hips should be raised by a pillow, for an hour if possible.

Some known causes of infertility in females are malnutrition, anatomical defects, hormonal imbalance, infectious diseases (such as chronic gonorrhea) or tumors.

Males account for about 40 percent of infertility problems. The usual cause then is the sperm—low in number, inactive or unusual in form. An allergic response between male and female is another possible cause.

Diagnosing and treating problems of infertility requires expert individual advice so I suggest you consult a gynecologist with special knowledge of infertility problems. Your nearest medical school may be a good referral source.

Sperm Count

Dear Dr. Schoenfeld:

I am a 26-year-old man and I wish to find out if I am sterile. I do visit my personal physician regularly for physical exams but each time I find myself too shy and self-conscious to ask him for that sort of test. Is there any place where someone like me can go and have this test professionally performed?

ANSWER: Why not ask your local medical association or nearest medical school to refer you to a urologist? He'll ask you to bring a fresh semen specimen to his office or have you produce one there. Then he'll examine your semen under a microscope to determine the number of sperm present and whether they are normally shaped and active.

Wear dark glasses and a false mustache if it'll make you feel better.

Wants Uterine Transplant

Dear Dr. Schoenfeld:

My girlfriend had a very unfortunate pregnancy before I met her. She had a Caesarian section and because of complications her uterus had to be removed. She does have her ovaries, however.

I would like to impregnate my girlfriend but obviously can't. Can you advise me on the pros and cons of her getting a uterine transplant or similar therapy?

ANSWER: I'm sorry to tell you that no operation for a uterine transplant yet exists. But adopting a child can be as fulfilling to a couple (and the child) as one born to them.

Adopted children even come to resemble their adoptive parents because of similar facial mannerisms and body movements.

7

Appearance

Male Genitals

Genital Size

Why should genital size be the greatest area of concern for men (and second greatest for women)? My guess is feelings of inadequacy focused on the genitals. It's easier to deal with a fixed fact, especially a physical part of us, than more nebulous aspects of our psyches. In effect, the writers seem to be saying, "If only I were larger all my problems would be smaller." This belief may be reflected also in man's interest in ever longer automobiles, larger TV screens, etc. Complaints about genital size are not restricted to citizens of the United States. The same kind of letter is received also from Canada, England and continental Europe.

Often writers will include their dimensions—with few exceptions they fall within the "normal" range of 5 to 6½ inches erect. Seldom do women write complaining of inadequate size in their men. The anatomical area of the problem seems to be within the skull rather than the genitals.

Whatever the cause of concern, there is no known method of increasing penis size after puberty. Before or during puberty, genitals and secondary sex characteristics such as facial and body hair and voice quality will be affected by hormone treatment. Such treatment, however, may close the growth centers of the long bones, thus stopping vertical growth. Vacuum type machines and stretching exercises are advertised in the underground press and elsewhere. No evidence exists for their effectiveness and they may be harmful.

Flaccid Confidence

Dear Dr. Schoenfeld:

For years now I've been embarrassed and laughed at in locker rooms, swimming pools, bathrooms, etc., because of the size of my prick. After intercourse, where I usually muster a barely adequate six inches, my prick shrinks down to one inch. One Inch! *I can't walk around all the time with half a hard-on (which brings it up to average size) and I'm well past puberty, so man, this is it! My question: In this age of such rapid medical and technical advancement what can I do to increase my prick size before I become so cock-conscious I'll be put in a loony bin. Help!*

Yours truly,
Tiny Tim

ANSWER: The use of the phrase "I usually *muster* a barely adequate . . ." is instructive I think. The writer thinks he is normal when erect but concerns himself with size when flaccid. He might have been somewhat relieved had he known differences between the length of flaccid and erect penises tend to be inversely proportional to the size of the flaccid penis.

The following letter describes one way a man can develop feelings of inadequacy about his penis.

Dear Dr. Schoenfeld:

My small son, now almost 4, seems to have inherited (from me, since his father doesn't have this problem) a shortage or imbalance of whatever it is that should make him completely and unconditionally the sex which he is. As with me, though I didn't realize it about myself until adulthood, his genitals are noticeably small for the rest of him—by two he had grown from 6½ lbs. and 19½ inches to I think about 30 lbs. and over 3 ft., but his penis had scarcely grown at all. And still hasn't. It's scarcely an inch erect and otherwise just a little peanut of a thing with almost no shaft (it's the head and ring of skin above it that stretch when he has an erection, but the rest is barely an eighth inch long). Well, it sounds as if I stand and stare at him which I don't and he's very unself-conscious about it of course, even proud—in all ways a thoroughly normal and hardy little boy except for this one hitch. Is my concern unreasonable? If not, can something be done now or later? I asked his pediatrician about it a few months ago and he shrugged it off with a chuckle and the remark that "big or little it'll cause enough trouble sooner or later."

A Common Fear

Dear Dr. Schoenfeld:

When at home by myself sometimes walking around in the nude or while taking a shower, I get an erection. What bothers me is when I think of going to a public place like a gymnasium to work out or a Turkish bath or some other place where I may be taking off my clothes. I worry that I may get an erection in front of members of my fellow sex in such a place. I know that all men get erections but should I be concerned about getting one in a public place?

How do other men feel about this? Does this ever happen to them and if so, does it bother them? Should I consider this a problem? I have never brought this up to anybody before because I thought I might be abnormal.

ANSWER: Your "problem" has worried almost all males at some point, especially younger men. But these fears are usually never expressed except, perhaps, to a psychiatrist.

Some solutions suggested by patients: jump into a cold shower, think of jumping into a cold shower, the face of your least favorite politician, remember the first time a policeman's flashlight shone into your car when you were making it in the back seat, recall a hospital or university cafeteria meal. The possibilities for turnoffs are endless. Another possibility is not to worry about it.

Thrown A Curve

Dear Dr. Schoenfeld:

If I should stand at home plate on a baseball diamond and look straight at second base, my erection would point to right field.

I have no performance problems to speak of and women are usually too occupied to even notice. But I'm very curious to know how common it is and whether it's a symptom of anything else. I've had this condition since puberty.

ANSWER: A list to right or left or a slight curve upwards is normal. More pronounced angles might be caused by chronic untreated gonorrhea, a rare condition known as Peyrom's disease or a congenital defect which prevents part of the skin from stretching. If you've noticed no variation since you reached puberty, there's no point in bending yourself out of shape further by worrying. You should consult a urologist though if you notice a change or encounter any functional difficulty. He could at least set your mind straight.

I'm very curious to know why a baseball diamond turns you on.

Dear Dr. Schoenfeld:

I was pleasantly surprised to see you used my question about angling erections. But as to baseball turning me on—I was merely making a graphic illustration. I don't even like *baseball!*

However, if I were to stand between the goalposts of a football field and look directly at Joe Namath . . .

Circumcision

A reader of *OZ*, the English underground newspaper, sent the following letter:

A bird I know recently pointed out to me that she prefers her boyfriends to be circumcised. She didn't go into any reasons except that "it was nicer."

From the point of view of cleanliness a foreskin is a bit of a nuisance and I might consider having it off if:

a) *there is more satisfaction without it and*

b) *it wasn't embarrassing to have it done 24 years late.*

Wouldn't people think it was abnormal or something?

ANSWER: Medical opinion on the advisability of routine circumcision is divided but all tests to date have shown no difference in sensitivity of the glans (head of the penis) or in satisfaction received in those circumcised or uncircumcised. Circumcision is a fairly common procedure in adults but this often seems to be a matter of social custom. The administrator of a local profit-making hospital told me of a recent case in which all the males in a family were circumcised simply because they qualified for the operation under welfare benefits. There are also cases when circumcision is a medical necessity.

Dear Dr. Schoenfeld:

I was circumcised as an adult, at the age of 24 in fact, some 14 years ago. I've never regretted it for a moment—nor, so she tells me, does my wife. But there is one danger I would warn of, by relating what happened to me. I went out on a date while the stitches were still in place, indulged in a very chaste good-night kiss on the steps of a woman's dormitory, had an erection that tore out a couple of stitches, and thereby managed to drench my trousers with blood. I've always wondered what the dry cleaner's staff thought when they had to clean those trousers.

For what it's worth, my own opinion is that I enjoy intercourse more because of being circumcised. Certainly it never occurred to me to be "embarrassed" about being circumcised as an adult.

Dear Dr. Schoenfeld:

How can a male determine whether or not he is circumcised? I am not sure about myself.

ANSWER: Buy the John Lennon–Yoko Ono album "Two Virgins." Neither John nor Yoko is circumcised.

Dear Dr. Schoenfeld:

If you have been circumcised, can you become uncircumcised through a skin graft?

One of my friends has been to Japan and he says there it is quite common for men who have been circumcised to get skin grafts.

ANSWER: Urologists, *moyles* and other proponents of routine circumcision cite as evidence for their beliefs the lack of penile cancer in Jewish men and the low incidence of cancer of the cervix in their wives. Circumcision prevents an accumulation of smegma, the cheesy substance beneath the foreskin thought to be a cancer-producing irritant. Routine circumcision also prevents tightening of the foreskin and certain penile irritations of infancy.

Opponents of routine circumcision point out that psychological effects on the infant are unknown. How does he perceive this attack on his genitals? No anesthetics are used and the baby almost always cries, though many physicians say the baby feels no pain (they mean it doesn't hurt the physician). Freud neglected this area, perhaps because he was a victim of the ritual.

Claims have been made that uncircumcised males are more sensitive, but the few objective tests made of this question have shown no difference in sensitivity.

My own opinion is that routine circumcision is unnecessary if mothers learn how to care for their infant sons. The foreskin should be regularly (and gently) pulled back from the head of the penis and accumulated smegma cleansed with soap and water. Boys should be taught this as a matter of personal hygiene. But even with scrupulous cleansing, some males will have persistent irritations and tightened foreskins requiring circumcision later in life. And circumcision in adult males requires hospitalization for several days.

Skin grafts to replace severed foreskins are possible; so is the graft of an entire penis (nonfunctional, except for the elimination of urine).

A physician proponent of routine circumcision said of his opposition,

"They are wrong as to the amount of the difference."

Or maybe it's much ado about little.

Unbalanced

Dear Dr. Schoenfeld:

Why does my left testicle persist in upsetting the symmetry of my body by hanging lower than my right?

ANSWER: Medical research has uncovered the fact that "lefties" predominate in this part of the male anatomy. The reason is obscure.

A blond communications coordinator believes psychological balance is more important.

Dear Dr. Schoenfeld:

I read the column in which one of your readers asked why his left testicle hung lower than the right.

If I remember correctly, this is so because the left spermatic vein empties into the left renal vein at a right angle whereas the right spermatic vein opens into the inferior vena cava at an acute angle.

The result is hydrostatic pressure greater on the left testicle than the right.

San Francisco M.D.

Wants to Be Uptight

Dear Dr. Schoenfeld:

Your recent remarks on testicles have stimulated me to ask for your comments on a related personal problem.

Normally my scrotum is completely relaxed, causing my testicles to dangle in an unsightly manner. Occasionally (and unpredictably) it tightens but usually not at an appropriate time, as when on view prior to intercourse.

Although this has vexed me since adolescence, I have never felt it was a great problem. This past summer, however, I had a couple of really great free beach experiences, during one of which I miraculously managed to keep a tight scrotum most of the time.

Since I now feel the free beach scene is the only beach scene worth making, I am writing in hopes you can suggest some treatment or exercise that would enable me to step onto a free beach next summer with a self-assurance I now lack.

ANSWER: The cremasteric muscles controlling the scrotum are not voluntarily activated, unless you can gain this control through yoga:

1) While lying in the sand have a friend run up, shriek loudly and throw ice water on your abdomen. When this has been done five or six times unexpectedly, you'll be ready for the next step which is:
2) While lying in the sun have a friend run up and shriek loudly, this time omitting the ice water. The desired reaction will be the same.
3) With a little imagination you can work out variations of this reflex conditioning so that even the thought of being on a beach can put you uptight. Or you can allow your body to do its thing, relax, dig the free beach scene and hang loose.

A New Wrinkle

Dear Dr. Schoenfeld:

Due to excessive masturbation using my thumb, I find I have one large crease and several smaller ones beneath the head of my penis, where the skin has been stretched.

I want to ask two questions: 1) Is my condition peculiar to myself or is it common among other males? 2) What the hell can be done about it, i.e., how can I remove the creases?

Please print this because I am slowly losing my mind with fear of embarrassment.

Sincerely yours,
The Crease

ANSWER: The chances of any condition being peculiar to one person alone are negligible. Since masturbation is not physically or mentally harmful, whatever its frequency, I suspect your anatomy is perfectly normal. Even if you do differ somewhat from most other males (and I doubt that), people won't wrinkle their brows over your creases.

If you haven't straightened this out by now, a visit to a free beach or a physician will help iron out the problem.

Overexposed

Dear Dr. Schoenfeld:

I have been an indoor nudist for quite sometime but have decided to take it all outdoors the rest of this summer since I've moved into a place with some privacy. Never having done any nude sunbathing before, I'm a little concerned.

For a first time exposure to the sun—should my genitals be exposed as long as the rest of my body? Also—if it occurs—what does one do for a sunburned cock?

ANSWER: Serious burns can result from exposing virgin flesh to the sun's rays. You should gradually increase the time you spend sunbathing beginning, say, with half an hour. But even experienced sun worshippers should be careful about not overdoing it. As a medical student in Miami I recall seeing a bright red mass of suffering flesh who had fallen asleep on the beach.

A number of commercial preparations are sold for the relief of mild sunburn. As for your specific question—it would make for an interesting television commercial, wouldn't it?

Breasts and Bottoms

Flattened Ego

Dear Dr. Schoenfeld:

I am just about to turn 13—in age but not in development. I'm almost as flat-chested as an 8 yr. old and it's so embarrassing. I can still wear undershirts when everyone else is wearing size 34 bras. But that's not the worst. It's when I'm swimming. My bathing suit shows just exactly how flat I am. So when I get out of water I have to cover up my chest so no one will think that I'm 8 instead of thirteen.

Please, isn't there anything I can do? I can't afford breast surgery and neither of my parents would even think of it. Aren't there any exercises I can do, or must I remain flat for life?

DOOMED

Dear Dr. Schoenfeld:

My tiny bosom throbbed with sympathy for the flat-chested girl who wrote to you. Her problem is more cultural and psychological than physical.

I used to feel inferior about my small breasts. Then I had babies and was suddenly well-endowed. So I nursed a long time and wore sweaters. The funny thing is, now that I've weaned and am tiny again, I don't feel bad any more because I know I CAN be big. I don't even like padded bras.

Pneumerology

Dear Dr. Schoenfeld:

I am 24 years old and for the past few years have been mildly embarrassed over the minuscule development of my breasts. I really look funny without any clothes on since otherwise I have a very feminine body. I went to see a doctor who said I was "normal," just very small.

While I understand that theoretically the size of one's breasts should not be significant, this problem detrimentally affects my sexual adjustment as a woman and underscores whatever feelings of inadequacy I carry around with me. Isn't there something which could be safely done about this?

Are silicone injections to increase the size of the bust safe? What is the best method of increasing bosom size? Don't tell me to try exercises—I have and they don't work.

I don't mind being smallbreasted but I do think a girl is entitled to at least a handful.

Sincerely,
Hope Chest

ANSWER: Silicone injections are still considered experimental procedures in this country. Even the experimental work was stopped for a time while the Food and Drug Administration investigated possible dangers.

Permission was recently granted to resume the experiments in all parts of the body except the breasts. Breasts were excluded because the presence of silicone makes it more difficult to feel possible tumors (though other, more accurate but less available diagnostic tests are possible). The FDA also worries about possible migration of the silicone, leaving, in a hypothetical case, one flat breast and one large buttock. At least one death has resulted from silicone incompetently injected by a person posing as a physician.

Silicone injections are useful in correcting certain cosmetic imperfections, though any experimental procedure may backfire, as indicated by the following letter:

Dear Dr. Schoenfeld:

Some time ago a doctor injected silicone into my nose just above the left nostril. Then the silicone started to come out.

I went back to the doctor and he removed an inch of hard white substance hanging out of a pore in my right nostril. He couldn't remove the rest of it.

Physicians who continue silicone injections to enlarge breasts maintain they are not dangerous and that their patients' improved mental health compensates for any possible hazard.

The officially approved method of breast enlargement involves placing silicone-filled plastic sacks under the existing breast tissue through surgical incisions. This procedure requires hospitalization and a cost of well over $1000, while silicone injections can be done in a physician's office and cost much less.

Exercises increase the size and firmness of the muscles beneath the breasts, making them more prominent, though the breast tissue itself is unchanged.

Now that I've answered your questions let me add my opinion: the size of a woman's breasts has nothing to do with her attractiveness.

Inverted Nipples

Dear Dr. Schoenfeld:

Could you please explain what inverted nipples are and what if anything, is the cure?

ANSWER: Inverted nipples turn in rather than out. The condition is rather common and should cause no concern unless it occurs after puberty. *But a nipple which inverts after puberty may be a sign of cancer.*

I've seen a picture of a suction device used to evert the nipples similar to those used to stimulate the flow of breast milk. Pregnancy may also cause them to evert. Some gynecologists suggest having a close friend suck inverted nipples at least once daily to cause eversion. Find someone trying to kick cigarette addiction.

Born Free

Dear Dr. Schoenfeld:

About the girls who want to know if they should wear a bra or not—no bra, if they follow certain rules. This means exercising the muscles that normally hold up the breasts. These you can find described in any beauty book that gives exercises for breast development.

Now if she starts wearing a bra all the time, sure enough every time she takes it off her boobs will sag to her waist. That's because the bra is doing the work of these muscles and the muscles stay underdeveloped. I'm very heavy breasted and haven't worn a bra in 10 years. I'm in my forties and short-waisted and my boobs are still well above my waist.

Also if these muscles are well developed when you are pregnant, nursing will not hurt their shape. My grandmother never wore a bra—she thought them sinful! I agree. About the only disadvantage of going without a bra and being heavy breasted is in running. Since I stay pretty much away from peace demonstrations, this hasn't been too much of a disadvantage.

Bras do the same to your breasts as girdles do to your stomach and rear end. Neither is desirable.

ANSWER: My secretary suggests a controlled experiment in which girls would wear bras with one cup. Only then will we know whether bras have any effect at all on breasts.

Printout

Dear Dr. Schoenfeld:

Certain female physical characteristics which really turn me on are just too rarely encountered in my experiences. I would like to find some way of predicting whether a given girl on just meeting (and fully clothed) may possess any or all of these luscious features:

1. *large nipples*
2. *normally erect nipples*
3. *perfect circularity of area surrounding nipples*
4. *definite tint of the surrounding circles, although rosiness or brownness itself is unimportant to me (I guess I mean here a definite contrast between area and skin tone)*
5. *large and protuberant (normally exposed) minor lips*
6. *moderate (at least not excessive) vaginal depth*
7. *minimal pubic hair*

Is there evidence of association of any of these features and some other characteristics which are more readily apparent on first meeting? An evidenced correlation of even plus or minus 0.50 would be a help with some of the above, since such would give odds of one in four that the prediction would hold.

Some probable associations have occurred to me but are of little practical worth, e.g. minimal pubic hair—Oriental race, more definite nipple areas—having had a child. These are little help since there are few Orientals in my locale and hassles with husbands or babysitters in the latter case.

If nothing else comes to mind, could you suggest sources where such information might be found?

ANSWER: Maybe there's a computer dating service listing the physical characteristics you desire. Readers may have other ideas. Aren't there other parts of women which interest you? Their heads, for instance?

Branded

Dear Dr. Schoenfeld:

After making love, my girlfriend and myself often leave "hickies" on each other. This sometimes proves embarrassing when we are around certain people, i.e., her parents. Is there any way to get rid of these telltale marks quickly when they appear? Or must we continue to wear turtlenecks?

ANSWER: "Hickies" or "monkeybites" are caused by blood oozing from broken capillaries beneath the skin surface. If you're tired of turtlenecks you can use body makeup or lower the pressure.

Bottom of Despair

Dear Dr. Schoenfeld:

I have a lovely body with a full, firm bosom, small waist and NO derriere. I can't wear pants or any clothes that are fitted in that area.

I have tried exercises specifically for the gluteal muscles for years to no avail. I feel I am almost becoming psychotic about this lack and am terribly jealous of any girl with a shapely bottom. I try not to let my husband see my nude body from the rear.

Perhaps silicone injections would help me. I know it's being done in my city but I don't know by whom.

ANSWER: It's true flat derrieres can become rotund with silicone injections.

On the other hand, perhaps your husband likes you exactly as you are and would be disappointed by any change. You'd better discuss the matter with him first.

Silicone injections in the buttocks seem to meet with FDA approval—even they have favorite parts.

A full-blown friend suggests getting a job as a stenographer. If that fails to round you out contact the nearest medical school.

Minor Hang-Up

Dear Dr. Schoenfeld:

I have a "condition" which seems to worry my husband more than myself. Ever since my teens my inner or minor vaginal lips have hung outside my major lips.

Because they are not tucked neatly within the major lips my husband believes this could indicate some disorder. What do you think?

ANSWER: There is nothing abnormal about the labia minora protruding through the labia majora. Why some of my best friends. . . .

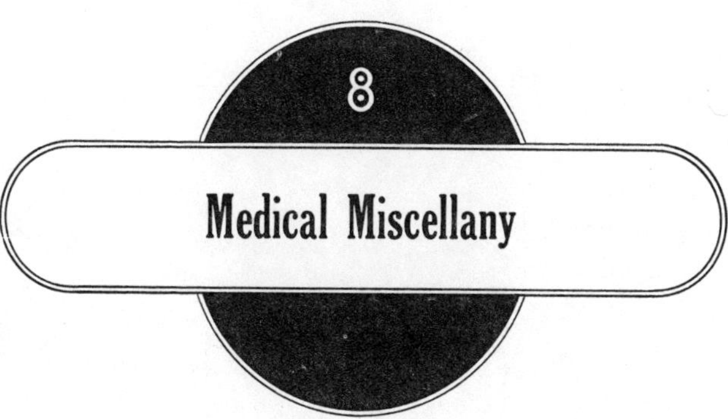

8

Medical Miscellany

Generic Drugs vs. Trade Names

Dear Dr. Schoenfeld:

I read an article recently about doctors prescribing drugs by brand names instead of their chemical names. Could you discuss this?

ANSWER: A common experience of patients is to find their pharmacy bills equalling or surpassing the physician's office fee. One reason for the high cost of prescriptions is the practice of designating drugs by their brand name rather than the generic or chemical name. A pharmacist usually must dispense the brand-name drug specified by the physician even though it may cost many times the identical drug produced by a lesser-known company.

Trade names are usually easier to remember than generic names. For example, chlorothiazide is the generic name of a common drug used in the treatment of hypertension (high blood pressure). Merck, Sharp & Dohme's chlorothiazide is called Diuril—shorter and reminding the physician that it functions as a diuretic or urine-producing drug.

The pharmaceutical companies employ "detail men" whose sole function is to promote drugs of the parent company by visiting physicians' offices and hospitals. Studies have shown that many physicians learn about new drugs not from scientific conferences or medical journals but from the detail men.

Drug companies spend huge sums on each of the country's 275,000 practicing physicians in order to sell their wares. Besides detail men, physicians are daily inundated with free drug samples and expensive multicolored advertising materials touting the benefits of one drug over another.

Despite huge promotional expenses, profits for the drug companies are higher than for any other major American industry.

The pharmaceutical industry claims prescribing by brand name rather than generic name insures drugs of better quality. Yet all drugs must meet United States Pharmacopeia (U.S.P.) standards. Following are prices to physicians of some commonly used brand-name drugs and the identical drugs produced by lesser-known companies. Prices in both categories would be higher to the consumer filling a prescription in his local pharmacy.

BRAND NAME	GENERIC
Penicillin tablets 400,000 units (Squibb) 100 tablets—$9.30	*Penicillin tablets 400,000 u.* 100 tablets—$1.50
Achromycin 250 mgm (Lederle) 100 capsules—$5.25	*tetracycline 250 mgm* 100 capsules—$1.55
Dexedrine tablets 5 mgm (SK&F) 1000 tablets—$22.60	*dextroamphetamine sulfate 5 mgm* 1000 tablets—$1.00
Nembutal 100 mgm (Abbott) 100 capsules—$2.65	*pentobarbital sodium 100 mgm* 1000 capsules—$3.35
Chlor-Trimeton 4 mgm (Schering) 1000 tablets—$21.00	*chlorpheniramine 4 mgm* 1000 tablets—$1.05
Miltown 400 mgm (Wallace) 100 tablets—$6.10	*meprobamate 400 mgm* 1000 tablets—$6.75
Meticorten 5 mgm (Schering) 100 tablets—$10.75	*prednisone 5 mgm* 1000 tablets—$3.95
Thyrar 1 grain (Armour) 1000 tablets—$13.25	*thyroid 1 grain* 1000 tablets—$1.45
Gantrisin 0.5 gm tablets (Roche) 1000—$24.75	*sulfisoxazole 0.5 gm tablets* 1000—$8.50

Sweden's pharmacies were nationalized on January 1, 1970. On that date, a state-controlled company bought all privately owned pharmacies in the country as well as two drug manufacturing firms owned by the pharmacists' association.

The goal of this move was to reduce drug prices and the number of drugs with identical uses.

Medical Ecology

Air Pollution Components

Dear Dr. Schoenfeld:

While driving in an open convertible on a Los Angeles freeway, eyes red and tearing, I wondered about the components of air pollution. What are they?

ANSWER: Substances generally considered to be the major air pollutants are as follows:

1. *Sulfur dioxide.* Irritates the respiratory tract. Largely produced by combustion of fuels. Through chemical reactions sulfur dioxide may be converted to sulfuric acid.
2. *Carbon* or soot. This is the visible pollutant found accumulating on windowsills. Soot may also carry cancer-producing agents into the lungs.
3. *Carbon monoxide.* Levels near freeways may be high enough to impair the mental efficiency of drivers. Blood levels of drivers involved in accidents are now being studied. Chronic cigarette smokers have even a higher level of carbon monoxide in their blood. The usefulness of blood donated by cigarette smokers may be reduced due to lowered oxygen transport capabilities.
4. *Carbon dioxide.* Causes "greenhouse effect" by admitting radiant heat from the sun while keeping convection heat close to the earth's surface. Because of the estimated six billion tons of increased carbon dioxide in the earth's

atmosphere each year, some scientists believe the earth's temperature is rising. One prediction is that the "greenhouse effect" will increase the mean annual temperature by 5.8 degrees F in the next 40 to 50 years.

5. *Hydrocarbons.* Found in petroleum products, coal and natural gas. At least one hydrocarbon, benzopyrene, is a known cancer-producing agent in laboratory animals. Soot may carry these compounds into the lungs.
6. *Nitrogen oxides.* Nitric oxide and nitrogen dioxide may pollute surface water as well as the skies. Ingestion of nitrates in the water may be harmful to man.
7. *Miscellaneous.* Fluorides, oxidants, ozone, peroxyacetyl-nitrate, aldehydes, lead, beryllium, arsenic, asbestos. Plus pesticides, fungicides and herbicides containing kerosene, sulfur, copper sulfate and cyanide.

Carbon Monoxide Poisoning

Dear Dr. Schoenfeld:

An average American automobile produces about six quarts of carbon monoxide per mile of travel. I can't help wondering if all that carbon monoxide in the air is helping to keep us insane enough to keep on putting it there.

Los Angeles M.D.

ANSWER: When carbon monoxide is inhaled, it combines with blood hemoglobin to prevent normal transport of oxygen to the body's tissues. Symptoms of carbon monoxide poisoning begin with headache, feeling faint, ringing ears, vomiting, cherry-red skin, dizziness and memory loss. Increased blood levels of the gas cause fainting, collapse, paralysis, unconsciousness and finally death.

Unvented heaters frequently cause accidental carbon monoxide poisoning deaths. And automobile exhaust fumes are often inhaled voluntarily to produce successful suicides. Recently a San Jose, California, couple was forced to leave their home because of illness due to dense carbon monoxide fumes arising from nearby heavy automobile traffic.

Ken Kesey believes the earth's atmosphere was once composed mostly of nitrous oxide (laughing gas). Maybe so. Certainly the quality of the air we breathe directly affects our heads, so wondering whether air pollution makes us weird isn't just idle speculation.

It's rumored that H-bomb father Edward Teller has designed massive air-purification systems for our cities. Twenty-story towers would suck in polluted air at one end and discharge pure clean air at the other. The pollutants would be collected and enough valuable minerals and gases extracted to pay for the maintenance of the purification towers.

Meanwhile the Peace and Quiet Party recommends you get out of the city next chance you have. Breathe deeply and notice the difference. Put some plants inside your house when you return and they'll help recycle your air.

Lead Poisoning

Physicians are becoming increasingly concerned with the effects of pollution on health. Excellent articles have appeared in the *Journal of the A.M.A.* and *Medical World News*. Recently the Bulletin of the Alameda-Contra Costa Medical Association featured an article on air pollution by John Rosen, M.D.

Speaking of lead poisoning, Dr. Rosen says, "With low level intoxication, we see weakness, lethargy, abdominal pain, headache, constipation, anorexia, pallor, and malaise. Lead is absorbed easily via the respiratory system . . . it does not have to be ingested. Samples taken from any ocean in the world now reveal presence of this element. It arises almost exclusively from our having added it to gasolines.

"Recent reports link lead intoxication with cancer of the kidney. What a price to pay for a quiet ride!"

Get the lead out!

Several cases of severe lead poisoning, including deaths, were traced recently to ceramic bowls and cups made with lead-based glazes. Lead is released when the vessels are used for cooking or for holding acidic fluids such as orange or apple juice. Some inexperienced potters like lead glazes because they produce a smooth finish but the resulting ceramics are highly dangerous when used for food or drinks.

On Latrines

City-bred people seeking a more healthful environment are often poorly prepared for life out-of-doors. Outhouses are sometimes seen perched over creeks or streams, for example.

I'll describe here a simple, fool- and flyproof method for building a pit-privy. First of all, don't contaminate water supplies. Latrines should be 100 feet from streams, springs or wells deeper than 20 feet, and 200 feet from shallow wells. If the ground slopes, build the latrine on the downhill side of the stream or well, unless you are aware of underground waterflow moving against the slope of the land.

A latrine should be at least three feet deep. Shallower holes will fill up faster, requiring more work in the long run (for the latrine). The edges should be raised slightly above the surrounding terrain and packed down. When possible, line the edges with tar or oil paper and tack the upper side of the paper to the wood planks which will cover the hole. If no lining paper is available, make sure there is a tight seal between the elevated rim of the pit and the covering planks. Don't forget to provide for a round or square hole in the boards covering the pit! A lid should cover this opening, preferably tied to the planks.

Refinements are building a seat for the structure and putting a building around it, i.e., a standard outhouse. But these are luxuries, unnecessary from a health standpoint. The important consideration here is to prevent flies from entering the pit.

An alternative method is to dig a long, fairly shallow, narrow "slit" trench. The excavated dirt is left by the side of the trench with a shovel nearby. Each time it is used, dirt is shoveled into the trench.

Dear Dr. Schoenfeld:

You described a way to construct a flyproof privy. The method seems simple, alright, but why must we hide a natural product of our bodies? Many of us left the cities so that we could live more naturally and free of uptight attitudes.

ANSWER: Disease prevention, rather than uptightness, is the reason for the proper disposal of human feces. Infectious hepatitis and typhoid fever are examples of diseases that may be transmitted in human feces even after symptoms have disappeared in the carrier. Amoebic and bacillary dysentery are commonly found in areas of the world where farmers use human feces for fertilizer. That's why travelers in the tropics are advised against eating uncooked vegetables. Flies have very hairy legs. If they light on our feces, they carry particulate matter to the next place they land—your macroburger, for instance.

Garbage Disposal

From the Loma Linda University School of Public Health, advice when garbage disposal is a problem.

> We recommend burying it in your own garden [says Karl C. Fischer, assistant professor of environmental health]. Just dig a long trench, about 18 inches deep, dump in the garbage and cover it up immediately with the dirt you dug to make the trench. Eventually, when that ditch is full, you plant a garden over it and dig another.
>
> In two years' time the buried garbage will be all rotted out. The tin cans, rusted out, will add iron to the soil. You do this instead of composting, and it will be the richest garden around.

Pinworms

Dear Dr. Schoenfeld:

I have a great lover who is perfect in almost every way, except for one very embarrassing problem—he keeps giving me pinworms.

I've gone to my doctor twice for a prescription, but this was getting expensive, so I started using a patent medicine. I'm too old-fashioned and embarrassed to discuss it at the source, and I am concerned about passing them on to my husband, who would be really turned off. I am taking so many showers that I'm turning into a prune. The main reason for writing is that I'm concerned about taking the patent medicine too often. Is there something more organic I could use besides eating garlic?

ANSWER: Pinworms are short, slender, white worms often found in children, but also in adults who share the same household. The most common symptom of pinworm infestation is itching around the anus, especially at night.

The itching is caused by female pinworms who move out of the intestines to lay their eggs on the skin around the anus. When asked why pinworms leave the intestines to lay their eggs, my medical school parasitology professor replied, "To get a breath of fresh air." Pinworms are transmitted by ingestion of the eggs. Besides itching, pinworm infestation may also cause mild abdominal pain, nausea, vomiting, diarrhea and loss of appetite. The diagnosis is made by applying a short strip of transparent cellulose tape to the anal area and examining the tape beneath a microscope for pinworm eggs.

Children (and adults) feel itchy, scratch, reinfest themselves or pass the eggs on to others. Treatment includes keeping the fingernails clean and short and washing hands with soap and water after bowel movements and before meals. Your friend (and his children) should follow the same procedures.

In addition to these preventive measures you or your friend should see your physician once more to get a prescription for medication. Unless he takes the medication as well, you will only be reinfected over and over again.

Garlic is very effective in preventing pinworm infestation as well as other communicable diseases by discouraging intimate physical contact. But it also has known therapeutic properties.

Dear Dr. Schoenfeld:

Your reader who is plagued with pinworms may be erroneously condemning her friend as the source of her discomfort. Infection with pinworms is such a common problem that it is virtually impossible to determine the source. Infection in adults is more likely in families with several children. My colleagues and I have found infection in over 70 percent of children in the 4 and 5 year age group in Los Angeles. Infection was present in 16 percent of adults in families with two or more children. We have made repeated efforts to eliminate pinworms from families, with only temporary success. Pinworm eggs float about in the air and can be found everywhere, even in chandeliers.

I am afraid that your recommendations for hygienic measures as part of the treatment will cause your reader an exercise in futility. Back in 1940 a team of investigators tested hygienic measures in an orphanage. They cleaned the rooms daily with soap and hot water, changed and sterilized bed sheets every day and required the children to take two showers a day and sleep in night clothes that also were sterilized daily. Special attention was directed toward keeping fingernails clean with nail brushes. After six weeks of this exhausting regimen the number of infected children had increased *by 13 percent. Unfortunately, this dramatic example was never widely publicized and textbooks and physicians have continued to recommend a routine that would frazzle the nerves of the most obsessive-compulsive housewife.*

The ubiquitous pinworm has us at its mercy. Thank goodness most of us don't *itch or even know we're infected.*

Sincerely,
Jerrold A. Turner, M.D.
Assistant Medical Director
Harbor General Hospital, L.A.
Assistant Professor of Medicine
and Medical Microbiology & Immunology
UCLA School of Medicine

Dear Dr. Schoenfeld:

I am a rather successfully analyzed 48-year-old former homosexual male (who practiced analingus promiscuously for nearly 2 score years) having been infected many many times with pinworms. Many times I got the prescription refilled, then a friend suggested plain yogurt, but I was not at the time interested in "health food faddists" so a few more years went by.

Then I thought I'd give the yogurt bit a go, which I did with amazing success. Every time I'd get infected I'd simply eat a couple of pints of the "no sugar added-plain" kind a day for a few days—less than a week and the itching would gradually go away (and I could no longer see any of them on my withdrawn finger). This worked for many years so I'm positive of its validity. Incidentally, I have children now and one of them has had them a time or two and it has worked with her also.

Ex-gay

Dear Dr. Schoenfeld:

Many years ago, when I discovered my 3-year-old son had lots of pinworms, I took him to the pediatrician and expected a prescription for some medicine. I was disappointed when I was told to give garlic instead, which I did.

I put garlic in soups and vegetables and in a very *short time the pinworms were gone, never to return.*

Dear Dr. Schoenfeld:

I was in Russia in 1918 when my brother-in-law returned from the German front. He had full stomach of pinworms. He went to an M.D. and was told: for three days you eat only salt herring and do not drink water *and in three days a ball of pinworms came out.*

Doctor:

Salted herring eaten for one day—nothing else—will clear up worms. Drink lots of water.

ANSWER: What! No sour cream?

Restaurants and Nude Feet

Dear Dr. Schoenfeld:

About restaurants that prohibit nude feet. Am assuming hygienic rationale: Are shoes more hygienic per foot?

ANSWER: Shoes are more likely to track in disease from the street than bare feet. Some restaurant owners cite health codes, but the truth is they just don't like barefooted customers.

I checked this out with the California State Department of Public Health and several local municipalities. No ordinance prohibits people from entering restaurants without shoes.

Dear Dr. Schoenfeld:

I'm a former partner in a restaurant. We were told to put up a sign forbidding bare feet by our insurance agent. Every day glasses or plates or both are broken. It is hard to get all the glass up.

Ladies tear their "best" hose every day. They want new ones. Dresses are torn, etc. Bare feet are prohibited to protect the people's feet and cut down on damages. Otherwise the small operator would be put out of business.

Believe me, we did not care what the customers wore or did not wear. They could have come without any clothes. We just wanted shoes on their feet—sandals, thongs or a shoe sole tied on with strings would pass the test.

ANSWER: Your reasons for banning bare feet are excellent. But why cite nonexistent health codes?

Crab Lice

Dear Dr. Schoenfeld:

Please, a short dissertation on crab lice, a by-product of my teenager's first year away from home. Can they be acquired, or re-acquired, by nonintimate contacts? Specifically—from toilet seats, bath tubs, bath towels, bedding, communal washing of clothing? How can they be vanquished?

MAMA

ANSWER: Crab lice or crabs can certainly be acquired through nonintimate contact. Bed linens, garments, towels or toilet seats can be sources of lice infestation. Treatment is simple and inexpensive—your pharmacist has several nonprescription medicines effective against crab lice. DDT should not be used—it won't kill crab eggs. The bedding, undergarments, etc., must be laundered at the same time, otherwise reinfestation may result.

How Often to Bathe

Dear Dr. Schoenfeld:

My old lady and I are having a huge hassle over what she calls my "unsanitary" body. I used to take a shower every day until I realized how stupid it was. Now I take a bath about once a month.

I don't see what's so unhealthy about it, but my old lady says it's unhealthy. Which of us is right? If she is, how often should I take a bath? Doesn't soap wash away the organic body oils?

ANSWER: Bathing is very healthy, natural and organic. In primitive cultures, the only people who don't bathe regularly are those who haven't ready access to water. I've noticed that people on communes with insufficient bathing facilities tend to have many skin infections.

How often you should bathe depends on your individual body chemistry, the amount of physical work you do, the weather, how close you want to be to strangers, and your old lady's sensibilities. Your friends and neighbors suggest twice a week for a start.

Dear Dr. Schoenfeld:

Your suggestion to the man who would rather not wash—that he should bathe twice a week—may be satisfactory to his "friends and neighbors" but for the sake of his old lady you should have recommended that he wash at least his genital area EVERY DAY.

On an active man, several day's accumulation of dirt, sweat, urine, sperm, vaginal juices, etc., etc., can make the pubic hair exude the most appalling odor and give the penis a dreadful acrid taste.

The Countess Tolstoy suffered for this precise reason when her husband decided to live like a peasant and refused to wash for weeks on end. And to this day women have some of their greatest pleasure spoiled because their men have some harebrained notion that it is sinful or unhealthy to wash.

Suffering In Berkeley

The Weaker Sex?

Dear Dr. Hip Pocrates:

In my school and, I'm sure, many other schools, we, the women, have been indoctrinated to think we are the weaker sex. We've been told that our only place is in the home because that is what our body was made for. I am very curious to know, can a woman, thru the same exercise as a man, attain the same physical strength? *This only seems logical to me that this would hold true. Free the woman of her false chains of weakness!*

ANSWER: Physical strength in both sexes can be increased through exercise but, in general, males have greater muscular strength. Women are stronger in other ways, for example they tend to live longer than men.

Most jobs today don't require brute strength. Females would be well represented in all professions if equal opportunities existed and if women chose to enter these roles. On the other hand, few jobs are as demanding, important and rewarding as properly caring for a home and family.

Many true biological differences besides sexual characteristics distinguish men from women.

Dear Dr. Hip:

You commented recently that ". . . few jobs are as demanding, important and rewarding as properly caring for a home and family."

Demanding? Yes! Important? Yes!!! Rewarding? Come on now! Let me give you one woman's reaction, which I'll put in a table because my work as a systems analyst tends to make me think that way:

INTRINSIC REWARDS

House & children

Lots; a child's first word; the humor of a child's delight in nursery rhymes; arranging a room to make it prettier; your husband cleaning up his plate and asking for more . . .

Job

A nice house if you earn the money; a raise if you do a good job (and sometimes even if you don't); the necessity for being well dressed; Paid-for trips to other places (for more interesting work); and you save lots of money by not having the time to succumb to the nation's abundance of come-on packaging, store display and advertising for worthless goods.

STATUS REWARDS

House & children

"Since we know you're home, won't you please give us a little time to do (a thousand worthy jimmy higgins jobs)."

Job

"We know you don't really have any time to spare, but we'd really appreciate your professional assistance on (a hundred interesting projects)."

GENERAL RECOGNITION

House & children

From a thousand editorial columns, psychologists, teachers, etc.: "If your children have problems and your house is a mess, it's clearly your fault and this is what you should do about it . . ."

Job

From your boss: "OK, maybe you goofed this time, but no one's perfect."—Maybe no raise this year. Firing? Not that often; I've met many more incompetent professionals and other employees than I've met incompetent mothers. From your profession or union: "This is the problem, now what are we going to do about it?"

Well, not to belabor a point any longer, I just don't think "home and family" vs. "job" comes out even. And believe it or not, I'm not even involved with women's lib.

ANSWER: This letter made me think of comparisons between medical specialists and general practioners. The practice of the GP is certainly as demanding and important as that of the specialist. But he has less status, money and recognition. "Just a housewife" is about the same as saying "just a GP." But I believe the family physician performs the most valuable function in medicine.

The Epidemiology of Earwax

Add to methods of tracing man's origins and movements across this planet the study of his cerumen, or in more prosaic terms, earwax. That's right, earwax.

Cerumen is either wet or dry, the type for each individual determined by simple hereditary laws. Wet cerumen is dominant over the dry type and heterozygous wet earwax (wet-dry parents) cannot be distinguished from homozygous wet earwax (wet-wet parents). Nor can homozygous dry earwax be distinguished morphologically from heterozygous dry earwax. The two types of cerumen differ not only in consistency but in color. Wet cerumen is light tan to dark brown in hue, while dry earwax is tan, light gray or black.

Cerumen types tend to follow racial lines. Orientals most often have dry cerumen while Caucasians and Blacks usually carry the wet type. Two faculty members from the Department of Preventive Medicine of the University of Mississippi's School of Medicine classified cerumen from 432 Choctaw Indians living in their state. Their findings were reported in the February 14, 1969, issue of *Science*.

Drs. Martin and Jackson drew their sample from inpatients, outpatients and ward visitors at a Public Health Service hospital and from Indians seen at home, field clinics and the annual Choctaw Indian fair. The authors found 79 percent wet and 21 percent dry in their sample. A previous study had found that the greater the proven mixture of Caucasian with Indian, the lower the frequency of dry earwax.

Drs. Martin and Jackson want to compare cerumen types of Choctaws from their state with those of Oklahoma Choctaws removed from Mississippi "by treaty" in 1830 (maybe they'll get another grant). Evidence is not yet conclusive but so far it seems that frequency of dry cerumen in Indians decreases as the distance from the Bering Strait increases. North American Indians are thought to have migrated to this continent across a land bridge now covered by the Bering Strait. A decreasing frequency of dry cerumen with increasing distance from Asia (remember that Orientals usually have dry cerumen) probably is a result of mixing with other races.

Peruvian Indians of pure blood, on the other hand, have a very low rate of dry cerumen, perhaps substantiating the belief they arrived in South America by boat rather than overland from Asia.

Anyway, higher truths often stem from humble origins so if this information seems irrelevant—stuff it in your ear

The American Way of Living Death

One of my first medical experiences was caring for geriatric patients at Fairmont–Alameda County Hospital in San Leandro, California. My chief was Dr. Fritz Schmerl, a noted gerontologist as well as an inventor (his bedside scale is widely used in hospitals for weighing patients unable to stand).

My special responsibility was Ward G. "G is for girls," Dr. Schmerl would say, his eyes twinkling. The average age of my "girls" was 83. Among my tasks at Fairmont Hospital was to give all the geriatric patients physical examinations, including pelvics for the Ward G patients. Many of them had been at Fairmont 10 or 15 years. We were to determine which patients could be transferred to the less expensive care given by nursing homes.

When payment for nursing home care was guaranteed by the government, a tremendous boom began in the nursing home industry. Between 1960 and 1965 the number of nursing home beds in California increased from 16,000 to 45,000. Almost all of these newly available beds were in profit-making nursing homes or "convalescent hospitals," to use the euphemism they prefer.

The invaluable experience I received at Fairmont Hospital under Dr. Schmerl later qualified me to head the Alameda County (Berkeley, Oakland) Health and Welfare Departments' Nursing Home Project, just after I received a Master's degree in public health. We were to suggest means of improving nursing home care and to try to insure that welfare patients were receiving at least minimal standards of care. My experiences that year convinced me the custom some tribes have developed—putting their aged infirm members out into the cold to die—is more humane than our system of nursing homes.

Unlike most general hospitals, 90 percent of nursing homes are operated for profit. Because geriatric patients are shunned by most health professionals, their care has largely fallen into the hands of people whose training and motivations differ greatly from those found in other health facilities.

The best nursing home care is given in institutions affiliated with churches or fraternal organizations such as the Masons. Good care in profit-making nursing homes is the exception rather than the rule.

Nursing homes were formerly converted boarding homes, which often provided newspapers with horror tales of trapped patients asphyxiating in winter fires. But the typical nursing home today is a fireproof structure of stucco, glass and plastic resembling a motel decorated in Miami Beach Modern. The resemblance to motels isn't accidental. Many nursing home chains have developed in the last ten years. The chain owned by Holiday Inns is listed on one of the stock exchanges.

When you enter a modern nursing home you'll see a lobby with motel-like furniture, plastic plants and a nursing station. Ladies dressed in white uniforms are in evidence, but few, if any, are trained nurses. They're nurse's aides, which usually means no training and payment of the minimum wage. Federal Medicare standards require a participating nursing home to have in its employ only one full-time RN or licensed vocational nurse. In California, a nursing home need have an RN on duty at all times only if the institution has 100 or more beds. CALIFORNIA HAS MANY 99-BED NURSING HOMES. Even these minimal standards are frequently violated because responsible regulatory agencies rarely have the personnel necessary to check for violations. Policing medical facilities shouldn't be required often, but nursing home operators are rarely health professionals.

It's far easier to finance the construction of a profit-oriented nursing home than a nonprofit institution because the Small Business Administration will guarantee 90 percent of the construction loan. Physicians are welcomed as investors because they assure a steady flow of patients. The number of nursing homes owned wholly or in part by physicians is a yet uncovered national scandal. These physicians, naturally, route their aged patients to their own institutions. Not uncommonly, a physician will spend an hour or so a week waving to thirty or forty patients in a nursing home while Medicare pays a nursing home visit for each of them. Standards of care would be higher if physician-owners actually supervised their nursing homes, but few are interested.

The term "convalescent hospital" implies the patients may return home someday, but this would be against the best business interests of the nursing home. Physical therapy, if available, is not included in the basic cost of care. Recreation usually consists of a TV set. Without physical or mental stimulation, the inevitable result is further deterioration.

From the standpoint of the nursing home operator, the best patients are those who require little care and do improve enough to go home. Should they require more care than they're "worth" they're sent off to a general hospital. When profits slip three recourses are available to the nursing home operator: 1) decrease the quality and quantity of food, 2) change bed linens less frequently, or 3) reduce the number of nurse's aides.

I picked up a nurse's aide recently hitchhiking in the rain. Our conversation confirmed that nothing had changed in the nursing home industry. She complained her feet hurt because no rugs were on the floors. Another nurse's aide, with the same institution for three months, had asked my passenger how to read a thermometer!

The poor standards of care, sterile environments and, most importantly, lack of concern and love make most of our nursing homes the American way of living death. No other industrialized country provides so pitiful a setting for the last days of its aged citizens.

Dear Dr. Schoenfeld:

I just read your article about convalescent hospitals. I am presently employed at ——— Convalescent Hospital in Los Angeles.

Since the State has cut down payments to nursing homes:

a) *our wages have been cut 10%. We make in most cases under $2.00 an hour.*
b) *we no longer have shower girls. Their duties were to shower each patient twice a week.*
c) *our hours have been cut down to 7 hours instead of 8 hours, plus do our own showers.*

Each patient should have a bed bath or shower each day, their teeth cleaned, hair brushed and dressed plus up in a wheel chair for 2 or 3 hours and back to bed. They are all entitled to this care. But under present working conditions the only ones that get any care are the ones who can holler if they get mistreated. The senile or bed-ridden patient gets practically no care at all.

ANSWER: Nursing homes (convalescent hospitals) operated for profit would have to shut their doors if they failed to make money. When income decreases the nursing home operator is forced to cut expenses. That translates to even worse care for his aged patients.

A health care facility should not be operated as just another business, but profits in the "nursing home industry" (the term they use) are squeezed from the bodies of Grandma and Grandpa.

Dear Dr. Schoenfeld:

The A.M.A. should long ago have built and supervised proper nursing homes with the money they've used through the years to fight health insurance and then Medicare (and now National Health Insurance, E.S.).

Most nursing homes are a disgrace and the medical profession, by its inaction, is responsible for their existence. Even strict government regulation wouldn't be as effective as regulation by doctors. That is, if doctors were honestly interested in the care of the aged.

Dear Dr. Schoenfeld:

The nursing home in America is too often a convenient place to abandon older relatives or people we don't want around us. The "rush" to get these people out of sight and mind causes a lack of concern for the places designed to keep older persons—the quality of nursing care given and the necessary "human touch" of real caring for the life of the person being overlooked.

Many people leave their aged parent(s) in a general or convalescent hospital and refuse to accept responsibility for their care for no better reason than that they don't want them around. The aged person has little to say about his future because the county assumes responsibility then—and it's off to the nursing home to stay. Shoving them in a nursing home is no solution, unless by making them feel unwanted, denying them a purpose or reason for living, and inviting emotional death is called a solution. There is little humanity, reason, love, or life in this system. It's downright cruel.

What is ironical is that this same "fate" will probably face every person in the future unless attitudes toward the aged and nursing homes change now.

Aunt Sadie

(Miami Beach) My Aunt Sadie has always seemed like a big woman to me. So I'm surprised even now when I stand next to her to find she's not so tall after all. I guess it's because she has such a hearty laugh and, when she's angry, a fiery stare that used to stop instantly whatever mischief her nieces and nephews were into. Uncle Harry is pretty quiet but I still remember the photo of him in the N.Y. *Daily News* centerfold standing over a holdup man he'd decked with a milk bottle from his grocery store. Now Aunt Sadie and Uncle Harry are retired in Miami Beach.

Aunt Sadie has a bit of arthritis so she's used to aches and pains now and then but recently she awoke with a pain in her back and right hip that just wasn't relieved by aspirin. The pain got worse and she called her internist but he was on vacation. His nurse recommended an orthopedist but when Aunt Sadie called his office she was told she'd have to wait five days for an appointment.

Aunt Sadie is a fairly stoical lady but the pain grew unbearable and finally Uncle Harry helped her into the car and they drove to Mt. Sinai Hospital's emergency room. They waited a long time because they have private medical insurance and, according to hospital policy there, a private physician had to be called in on the case. The orthopedist who finally arrived was from the same office which couldn't book an appointment for Aunt Sadie until the following week. Well, that's understandable. Calls from an emergency room demand immediate attention.

After examining Aunt Sadie briefly the orthopedist decided X rays were needed and that's kosher too. But he told her she'd have to go to *his* office for the X rays. So Uncle Harry helped Aunt Sadie into the car and they drove to his office for the X rays. He told her she had a pinched nerve and would have to be hospitalized so they drove back to Mt. Sinai where she was placed in traction.

Now perhaps this physician has X-ray facilities superior to Mt. Sinai's but Aunt Sadie suspects he just wanted the insurance money. She always was pretty hip. After the first week in the hospital she wasn't even sure who her doctor was because the orthopedist shared his office with several other physicians and a different one visited her each day. One morning the physician she thought was in charge of her case was making teaching rounds with some residents. Aunt Sadie asked him a question about her X rays. He replied he hadn't seen the X rays and walked out of the room.

A few days later a nurse told her orders had been received to take her out of traction. Several days after that she telephoned the man she guessed was her physician and asked when she might go home. "First we'll take you out of traction," he said.

"But I've been out of traction three days," she replied, in her old fierce style, I imagine.

So Aunt Sadie signed herself out of the hospital and went home. She thinks something is wrong with our system of medical care.

Tear Gas and Mace

Dear Dr. Schoenfeld:

While watching the action attending the occupation of People's Park, I received several mild doses of tear gas. The result seems to be a considerable lessening of congestion in my sinuses though I suffer from chronic sinusitis.

Do you recommend this treatment?

ANSWER: Two types of tear gas were apparently used during the Berkeley People's Park crises, CN and CS. Technically, they are not gases but solids dispersed as aerosols.

CN or chloroacetophenone ($C_6H_5COCH_2Cl$) is a fast-acting irritant to the eyes and upper respiratory passages which was invented at the end of WWI. According to *Chemical and Biological Warfare* by Seymour Hersh, the official military manual TM3–215 states:

> In higher concentrations it is irritating to the skin and causes a burning and itching sensation, especially on

> moist parts of the body. High concentrations can cause blisters. The effects are similar to those of sunburn, are entirely harmless and disappear in a few hours. Certain individuals experience nausea following exposure to CN.

CS or o-chlorobenzalmalanonitrile is said to have been developed by the British in the 1950s. The *S* means "super" and its formula is $C_1C_6H_4CHC\ (CN_3)$.

> CS produces immediate effects even in low concentrations . . . The onset for incapacitation is 20 to 60 seconds and the duration of effects is 5 to 10 minutes after the affected individual is removed to fresh air. During this time the affected individuals are incapable of effective concerted action. The physiological effects include extreme burning of the eyes accompanied by copious flow of tears, coughing, difficulty in breathing, and chest tightness, involuntary closing of the eyes, stinging sensations of moist skin, running nose, and dizziness or swimming of the head. Heavy concentrations will cause nausea and vomiting in addition to the above effects.
>
> TM3–215

On May 20, 1969, a military helicopter sprayed tear gas over the Berkeley campus of the University of California. The gas, probably of the CS type, enveloped Cowell Memorial Hospital and drifted up to the Strawberry Canyon Recreational Area, affecting small children and their mothers. The following instructions for treatment of exposure to tear gas were prepared by Henry Bruyn, M.D., then director of Cal's Student Health Service:

> *Slight-Moderate Exposure*
>
> EYES—expose to fresh air. Do not rub.
>
> SKIN—keep dry for 4–6 hours. If the skin is wet, shower with soap.
>
> NASAL DISCHARGE—will subside rapidly without treatment.

SHOES—should be washed with a sponge or cloth.
GREASE OR OINTMENT—should NOT be used before or after exposure, otherwise the gas particles will cling to the skin.

Heavy Exposure (powder will be visible on the clothes and body)

EYES—large amounts of plain tap water. Burns of the cornea are possible so eyes should be checked by a physician. Recovery takes about 2 weeks.
SKIN—water increases the stinging but helps prevent burns.
HAIR—should be thoroughly washed.
CLOTHES—should be washed with a detergent.

Medical personnel may be affected by a patient's skin, hair and clothing. Victims of a severe tear gas attack should, if possible, remove their clothes and shower before entering a treatment area.

Tear gas may linger for long periods on cloth and paper. A visit to Cody's Bookstore on Haste and Telegraph caused my eyes to tear a week after one of Berkeley's tear gas episodes.

I can't really recommend tear gas as treatment for chronic sinusitis, but I'd like to know if other readers had similar effects. Perhaps leaders in future demonstrations will all have postnasal drips and wave handkerchiefs instead of flags.

Benefits of Riot Gas

Dear Hip:

Since every soldier in Basic Training at Fort Jackson, S.C., goes through the CBR (Chemical, Biological, Radiological) drills, I thought you might find it interesting that, yes, a dosage of riot gas works wonders for the sinuses. At the time I went through the "exercise" I had a beautiful case of what the military calls URI or upper respiratory infection. Couldn't breathe, lot of mucus, teeth aching, sore throat, the whole body aching. When I came out of the riot gas, oh lordy, it was all gone. See, the Army is *concerned about the health of its soldiers. But like God, they work in mysterious ways.*

Pax Vobiscum

Self-Preservation

Dear Dr. Hip:

Now is the time for all good scholars to go back to those "hallowed halls of academe." Many of us are no longer afraid of tests, profs or studies—it's the clubs, Mace, and tear gas that scare the hell out of us. How about a short course on self-preservation?

What are the latest remedies for a cracked skull, a Maced face, tear-gassed eyes or bird-shot buttocks. Also, what about some hints on protecting ourselves. Should I still be carrying Vaseline in my lunch bag?

ANSWER: Head injuries should always be evaluated by a physician. Even though no external wound is evident, serious damage may result from a club to the head. Danger signals are nausea, vomiting, headache, dizziness or blurred vision. Gunshot wounds, of course, also require immediate medical care.

The best treatment for Mace or tear gas is cool tap water and fresh air. Leave the petroleum jelly (Vaseline) out of your lunch bag. Rather than protecting you, the jelly will trap tear gas particles.

Mace

An editorial in the British journal *New Scientist* of June 20, 1968, comments on a study of Mace by Drs. Seever, Villarreal, and MacLeod of the University of Michigan's Department of Pharmacology. Following research on monkeys, the authors concluded that three provisions were necessary for the safe use of Mace:

1. The recipient must be alert, in possession of his normal protective reflexes such as blinking, closing his eyes, holding his breath and turning away from the spray.

2. The spray should be aimed at him from far enough away to allow these reflexes to come into play.
3. Spray must be limited to the shortest time demanded for the Mace to incapacitate the victim effectively.

The editorial continues, "According to the report severe long-term and maybe permanent damage could occur to the eyes if the corneas are exposed directly to Mace in liquid form. This could happen if Mace was discharged into the face at very close range, if large amounts were sprayed into an incapacitated person's face, or if large amounts were discharged in a small space, such as a car." The editorial goes on to ask if we are really to believe that police carefully assess the alertness and reflexes of all "recipients" before launching their attack from a "safe" distance and for the shortest time demanded for effective incapacitation of their victims. The editorial concludes with the following sentence: "Mace is a dangerous damaging weapon and it should be proscribed."

First aid for Mace victims should include copious amounts of running water in the eyes or wherever contact has occurred.

Medical Records and Government Spies

The relationship between patient and physician has always been the integral component of the practice of medicine. Medicine, we were told as students, is both an art and a science. The wise physician knows healing requires more than prescribing medications or maneuvering surgical tools. Scientific studies confirm that half or more of visits to family physicians or internists involve complaints for which no physical basis can be found. Not that the distress felt by the patient is any less real than if a definitive physical cause could be discovered. Certainly the acute pain of a headache caused by nervous tension can be as severe as one produced by a brain tumor.

Regardless of the type or level of training received by the healer, whether he be Mexican Curandero, African medicine man or Park Avenue superspecialist, the treatment process more often than not involves a "laying on of hands" and faith in the practitioner. Throughout the long history of the practice of medicine, one concept has remained unchanged—at least until recently. Confidences expressed by patient to a physician are inviolate. The ethical practice of medicine demands that what transpires between patient and doctor shall not be made known to any other person unless so requested by the patient. Legal statutes occasionally conflict with this concept but physicians have chosen to face prison terms rather than disobey what they know to be a higher law.

Sometimes a doctor is powerless to protect the privacy of his patients even though the law may coincide with his ethical standards. Surely it is not a new or particularly startling observation that governmental investigative agencies will employ extralegal methods to obtain information they believe necessary for internal or external security. To cite one such case, after the Free Speech demonstrations, I examined several patients in the emergency room of Berkeley's Herrick Memorial Hospital. Four years later, my brother underwent a security investigation prior to his induction into the armed forces. Investigators read him the names of the demonstrators and asked if he knew anything about them, their examination or the Free Speech incident. He didn't, of course, since he was attending medical school in a distant city at the time.

Recently, three cases involving patient-doctor confidentiality have become important news issues. The first occurred when the American Medical Association urged physicians through its weekly newspaper and two specialty medical journals to help capture a young woman indicted for conspiracy to transport illegal explosives across state lines. Since she has chronic severe acne, one of the "wanted notices" was placed in the *Archives Of Dermatology*.

The second case involved Mrs. Dita Beard, the celebrated lobbyist for International Telephone and Telegraph Corporation. When columnist Jack Anderson published a memo from Mrs. Beard alleging a $400,000 payoff to scuttle an antitrust suit against the giant ITT conglomerate, Mrs. Beard disappeared and was later found in the cardiac ward of an osteopathic hospital. Her illness was said to be angina pectoris, a condition which can vary from mild twinges of pain to a debilitating sickness. Usually there are no detectable clinical findings except the patient's complaints. Several lay people told me their impression based on newspaper accounts was that she was gravely ill. I did not make such a diagnosis. What interested me more was the spectacle of her physician testifying about her health to a Senate investigative committee. If, as he said, she was subject to "distorted and irrational" behavior, she could no more competently grant permission for him to speak publicly of her health and behavior than if she were seriously ill with a cardiac condition. I wonder how many physicians felt, as I did, a deep sense of revulsion as the woman's alleged medical history was used in an attempt to explain away an incident causing great embarrassment to the present administration.

The third case was the Ellsberg psychiatrist break-in, perpetrated by the same criminals responsible for Watergate. Most thefts of medical records, of course, have never been reported.

Judging from its silence on this issue, the American Medical Association seems to have little interest in the sacred relationship traditionally existing between patient and healer.

The Old and the New

Dear Dr. Schoenfeld:

Do you know of a medical school that isn't bogged down in tradition and doesn't prepare doctors to enter a "nice lucrative practice in suburbia," but does prepare them to deal with today's problems?

ANSWER: Take a look at and speak with some of the new medical students, interns and residents. They're more concerned with the world around them and medical schools are responding to these concerns. Times have changed since this statement by Donovan F. Ward, M.D., a recent president of the A.M.A.:

"We have no choice except to stand firm in our unshakable belief that if we have been right in the past, we are right today and we shall be right tomorrow."

Peace and Quiet Party Bulletin:

Heard from San Francisco attorney Vasilios Choulos:

"YOU ARE WHAT YOU HATE."

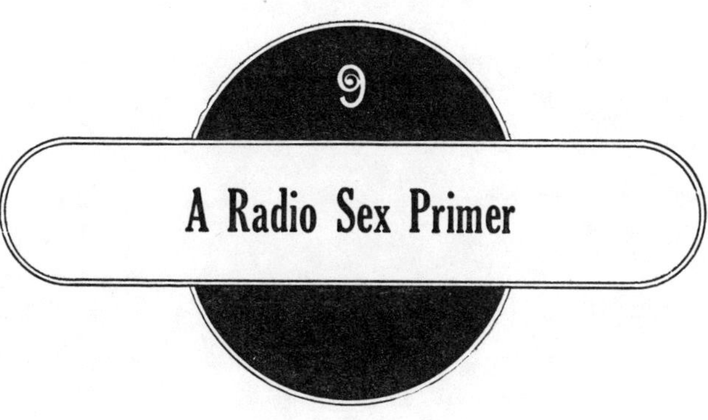

9

A Radio Sex Primer

A Radio Sex Primer

Introduction

I used to do a live weekly medical question-answer type radio program in San Francisco. One Sunday night my guest was Margo St. James, formerly the *Realist* nun and ex-hooker.

Paul Krassner, editor of the *Realist*, did a special three hour guest appearance just before my program began. He'd just been fired from another San Francisco radio station, probably because the previous week Margo dropped by his show and when asked what she recommended people do that Halloween night, replied "Give head." Oral sex, that is. Paul gave station breaks like, "This is the station that blows your mind."

My program with Margo St. James also dealt largely with oral sex. A transcript was made thanks to the interest of the Federal Communications Commission, an interest aroused by an attorney who claimed he dialed my program by chance while in the company of his wife. So offended were they at hearing real talk about oral sex on the radio they couldn't dial another station or switch their radio off entirely. The attorney's letters of complaint to the FCC caused a good deal of activity around the station for many months.

Metromedia sweated for a year over the station's broadcast license, worth millions of dollars. We submitted many letters to the FCC from medical experts supporting us and the idea of frank talk about sex on the radio. The station wasn't penalized.

That's the background to the following contribution to radio history and well-being:

Transcript of Program, KSAN–FM, Nov. 7, 1971

DOCTOR: Last week we were speaking with a lady from a Berkeley clinic for treating sexual problems. We were speaking with this lady who is a "practical sexual therapist," and what she does there is to treat sexual hang-ups very directly. This week, I thought we would talk not about sexual hang-ups but about more or less normal sexuality—whatever that is. We're going to talk with Margo St. James about ways of making it a bit better. I guess that's a way of capsulizing what we're going to be talking about: making good things better.

Margo, can you tell us what you are? You have something to do with exercise and I wonder if you could tell the listeners what kind of exercises and how long you have been doing this. Maybe, by way of introduction, I should say that Margo was the *Realist* nun–for those of you who have been following *Realist* magazine—and she used to do things that were then thought of as outrageous. I guess people would still be outraged by a nun seeing someone off at an airport and suddenly falling into a heavy clinch.

Margo, what—you say you're an exercise specialist —what was the title you told me?

GUEST: I said "sexercise" and—

DOCTOR: Actually, there is a book out called *Sexercises* and it's not bad.

GUEST: I'm just stealing their word.

DOCTOR: You're a sexercise therapist, is that right?

GUEST: You could—well, I'm into, I work for pussy power.

DOCTOR: Pussy power. What is, ah, how would you define that?

GUEST: Pussy power is woman's sexual potential. It's infinite actually, I think.

DOCTOR: Well, what's wrong? Do you think this potential isn't being exercised, so to speak?

GUEST: True, yeah. The frozen pelvis abounds in this country; and they just shed their girdles, this last generation, and the women's muscles are still unworked. Very few women have what men refer to as "snappy pussies." What do you call 'em on this show, anyway?

DOCTOR: Well, on this show we'd probably say, we'd probably say that you believe most women don't have the full development of the muscles which surround the vagina.

GUEST: Right. I find that some of my friends don't like to be, being thought of as uptight, so they walk around hanging out all the time or just in a loose position, and . . .

DOCTOR: Do you walk around all the time clenching those particular muscles?

GUEST: Yeah, that's a good idea. I mean to do it, relax it and do it, and tense, release, so that you become aware of where they are and you can move them at will whenever you would like. And there's not only just one set; there's two sets. And one has to exercise so that you can hold the surrounding ones tight and do the push, pull number on the inside, so that if you're practicing a type of Tantric sex you can lie still, the man can lie still and you can just massage him with your vagina.

DOCTOR: What kind of exercises would a lady do to strengthen the outer muscles?

GUEST: Well, I think the best thing for her to do, of course, is practice alone at first, and insert a finger so she can tell when those muscles are closed, when they're tight and when they're not; and do this until she reaches a point of awareness so that she can tell just by thinking about that muscle what it's doing.

DOCTOR: Right. If there are any ladies now out there, if they want to they could do that, I guess.

GUEST: Right. Yeah.

DOCTOR: Well, how would you describe how to clench these muscles? Just by their feelings . . . ?

GUEST: If before you pull "up" you could think "up"—the word "up" and pull everything up from there.

DOCTOR: Some people suggest that the way to do this, to begin to exercise these muscles is by making believe you're trying to avoid urinating. Would that do it?

GUEST: Well, I think that might work, sure.

DOCTOR: I mean, I'm just passing on things reported to me 'cause I mostly—I'm speaking from secondhand experience; speaking from the research of my research assistants.

GUEST: Well, I think that would work, and then on the release you could do it in the opposite way—it would be like trying to urinate, and this would be the push from the inside muscle, you know. I think if you tried to urinate that that would work that muscle.

DOCTOR: Some people have also said you could exercise these muscles, or one set of the muscles, by acting, straining down, as if you're going to move your bowels, but, of course, not doing it.

GUEST: Yeah, right.

DOCTOR: Which set of muscles do you think this would exercise?

GUEST: Well, that would be the inner ones, I think. The push is bearing down, like in childbirth, you know, same type of thing. And if you, but it's very difficult to, when one first discovers that there are two sets there, separate the two and get them to move separately—individually—that's what's necessary to have a true "snapper."

DOCTOR: How long do you think a woman would have to exercise to develop these muscles . . .

GUEST: I think, if it were done diligently, every day, whenever they're driving around in the car or when they're

—you can do it, see, you can do it and no one knows you're doing it. . . .

DOCTOR: A lot of girls have told me that they do it waiting for buses.

GUEST: Right, right, sure. Kill some time and just see how many times you can do it consecutively in tense—release—tense—release, and sometimes only two or three times, and pretty soon, in a few days you're up to 12. In three weeks you should be capable of doing any number and in rhythm, in time to music, even.

DOCTOR: Well, what advantage does this have?

GUEST: What—ah, the advantage is, it increases one's own enjoyment. It, you know, it gets you more into the oneness thing that's . . .

DOCTOR: So it's not only good for the male, but . . .

GUEST: Right—oh, it's potentially good for the female and I wasn't thinking of doing it for the male at all. It's for the enhanced enjoyment of the female. Because that area has been like dead for years, you know, throughout the Victorian scene, and people block out that part of their body. Many people I know aren't even alive from the waist down; they feel nothing. They can't move their bottom around at all.

DOCTOR: That's another kind of exercise now—what about pelvic movements? Even though someone might be able to do all kinds of snappy gyrations within, some people also have a frozen pelvis. Now, dancing, certain kinds of dancing, would help I would think.

GUEST: Right. Well, like the freak dancing, psychedelic dancing's good, you know. It'll get you to lose your self-consciousness and overcome your awkwardness just by getting loose and swinging your arms around and hips and shoulders and dancing with your elbows and everything into it. Then being able to stand still and just move one part of your body by itself helps you become aware of where that is.

DOCTOR: I know that you do a lot of running also. You were, in that race—what's the name of that race where you run across the City into Golden Gate Park?

GUEST: The Bay to Bridge race. And the Dipsea race, also. I do both of those every year. I love to run, I feel very free when I'm running. I especially like running on the beach in front of your house.

DOCTOR: Um . . . I like it, too. I like to see you running down the beach.

GUEST: I'd like to be able to run naked on your beach, but so far I haven't done it.

DOCTOR: There are people there with telescopes who get uptight at things like that.

GUEST: Yeah.

DOCTOR: But I wouldn't care.

Commercial—Judie Sill

Public Service Announcement—Speed

Public Service Announcement—Weed

DOCTOR: So far, you've been talking about exercises for ladies. What about men?

GUEST: Well, I think one of the things a man could do is try to let ladies be and regard them as human beings, and not get into the grasping, desirous, lecherous, lusting attitude that's such a turn-off in a lot of cases.

DOCTOR: You mean, like someone who's not so—

GUEST: Who's more interested in being a real friend and communicating instead of dominating, and who—

DOCTOR: You mean responsive to the other person.

GUEST: Right. Allowing the—other person's responses to trigger some of his own, you know, and becoming a one, a oneness, that is—

DOCTOR: But, that isn't exercise.

GUEST: Well, it is. It's an exercise in attitude.

DOCTOR: It's a mental exercise. Yeah.

GUEST: Well, men really aren't—

DOCTOR: We don't *have* to talk about physical—we're not going to restrict this to physical exercises.

GUEST: Well, let me put in this one little thing anyway. You know, men usually do the pelvic number anyway; they can go back and forth pretty good, but they can't go sideways too well.

DOCTOR: Especially not in that position.

GUEST: Right. And they should practice touching lightly things, y'know, even on themselves—just touching as light as they can with their fingers to develop a more gentle touch, which will turn the ladies on a little more. Most men are too heavy-handed and, you know, that's to be expected.

DOCTOR: Oh, why?

GUEST: Well, their type of work, and they don't really have that much contact with—with ladies who say what they like.

DOCTOR: It's really hard for people to communicate these things in words.

GUEST: Well, they're nonverbal.

DOCTOR: Even people who have been together for years. This is KSAN-FM, San Francisco, and it's 9:29. We're speaking with Margo Saint James, and we're talking about sex. The phone number here is 986–6244 if you have any questions to ask of Margo or myself or of Bonnie. We have here a typical suburban housewife, a lady who lives in Marin County. Her name is Bonnie.

ENGINEER: Don't give my name!

DOCTOR: Oh, all right.

ENGINEER: This is free, revolutionary free radio.

DOCTOR: Oh.

ENGINEER: And we can't have it known that people like me are living in the suburbs.

DOCTOR: Well, okay. We like to get representatives from various groups in the population, and so if you have any questions for Bonnie, who is a—how would you describe yourself, Bonnie? Let's go to the phones. Hello, you're on the air.

MALE CALLER: Oh, uh let me get my radio.

DOCTOR: Okay.

MALE CALLER: Right. You were talking before about loosening up the lines of communication. It's kinda hard to talk, you know, but I really feel that this would be an appropriate time for me to find something out here.

DOCTOR: All right. What would you like to find out?

MALE CALLER: About cunnilingus.

DOCTOR: What about it?

MALE CALLER: Is the woman there—I forget her name.

DOCTOR: Her name is Margo.

MALE CALLER: Margo, what is it that's really the best way to get that real good, y'know, relationship in that act, so that I can really know that I'm getting the full amount out of it, cause I feel I'm not now.

GUEST: Well, how do you do it? Do you do it sixty-nine or one at a time?

MALE CALLER: Ah, well, it's kinda hard; sometimes it's sixty-nine and sometimes it's not, y'know; and I kinda have to get into it so that I can really get her interested in the same way, you know, so that she just doesn't stay off to the side; and I feel if I could, you know, manipulate it in the right way—because sometimes I feel that she's riding wrong on me and she's not really into it, like she's detached or something, you know, and maybe I could do something to turn her on more.

GUEST: Well, you're confusing me. I don't know if you're talking about balling or eating.

MALE CALLER: Yeah, right, that's what I'm talking about—eating it.

DOCTOR: It sounds as if he wants to know, when he has a feeling that his lady isn't really into it, he wants to know what he should do.

MALE CALLER: And then she'd ball me back.

GUEST: Oh, okay. Okay. I think one of the more valuable techniques inasfar as keeping a woman in condition to enjoying a full vagina is the insertion of a finger at the same time that you're giving her head.

MALE CALLER: Right.

GUEST: And, you know, don't be too vigorous.

MALE CALLER: I know, I know. You've got to watch the teeth.

GUEST: Well, yeah, and stubble if you have—if he shaves.

MALE CALLER: Oh, yeah. Well, I do have a moustache.

GUEST: Well, a moustache is fine.

MALE CALLER: Okay.

GUEST: I think if you practice in the Queen's position, which is you lying between her legs on your stomach . . .

MALE CALLER: Uh huh.

GUEST: . . . that you could concentrate fully on the spot and she could concentrate on the same spot—two people concentrating on the same spot should get better results . . .

MALE CALLER: Yeah.

GUEST: . . . if you're having trouble that way—with her attention wandering.

MALE CALLER: Right. Those were a couple of good pointers, definitely.

GUEST: Try to create a vacuum with your mouth.

MALE CALLER: Yeah.

GUEST: Not a very big vacuum; just a slight one.

MALE CALLER: Yeah. I've already done that with my chin, to a certain extent.

GUEST: Well, your chin isn't too good to use, especially if you shave, and it's bony, and it's . . .

MALE CALLER: That's the trouble, yeah. So the lips are always better then.

GUEST: Yes. It's not too good to move your head around too much, unless she's really in heavy throes of passion, and then you can get more excited and more vigorous, but—

MALE CALLER: Um hmm.

GUEST:—keep it gentle.

MALE CALLER: Yeah. I'll definitely have to try that suction, too, that way.

GUEST: Yeah, and exercise your tongue so it doesn't get tired, so you can do it for at least a half an hour, y'know.

MALE CALLER: Yeah, right. Hey, thanks a lot!

GUEST: You're welcome.

MALE CALLER: Okay, bye, bye.

DOCTOR: Hope you can use that information to good advantage. . . . Margo, you just told him—he should exercise his tongue—how do you recommend he exercise his tongue?

GUEST: Well, I think that every morning after one brushes his teeth—men and women both—just stick your tongue out; look at it, y'know; curl it around; move it; make sounds with it, different sounds; and feel the inside of your mouth all over with your tongue; y'know, just—

DOCTOR: Well, I was wondering if you meant like when people start to play the piano, they do exercises—

GUEST: With their fingers.

DOCTOR: With their fingers, right, so I thought maybe you meant people should move their tongues to each side of their mouths, twenty times, three times a day. . . .

GUEST: Right. When you're driving down the road for two minutes, y'know, on your way to work, do it, and it's about, oh, the length of one record, say. If you happen to have your radio on. Do it in time to the music. And, after a while, you can do it for an hour at a time without even getting tired in between.

DOCTOR: Okay.

GUEST: It's just kind of like tickling the gums at the back top of the teeth—that's the spot—in fact, it might even tickle so much you have to stop.

DOCTOR: Let's take another call. Good evening, you're on the air. Hello.

MALE CALLER: Okay. I have a question about what Margo said about using a light touch for men. Some of the women I've been with say that they really like a heavy touch.

GUEST: Well, they do like to be dominated—feel dominated sometimes, tell you if they want it harder, but lots of times it's better to start out light.

MALE CALLER: Right.

DOCTOR: Different people just have different preferences—

I know what you mean. One likes a very light, sensitive touch. And then, with another lady with different preferences—ah, you're in trouble for a little while.

MALE CALLER: Right. Thank you very much.

DOCTOR: Margo, we were talking about exercises before, and you mentioned you wanted to talk about something else besides these specific exercises.

GUEST: Yeah. Complaints that I hear from men who are reluctant to participate in oral sex—they like to receive but they don't like to give—most of their complaints are that it smells bad to them.

DOCTOR: Well the lady must have an infection then, if that's true.

GUEST: Usually, yes, that's the case.

DOCTOR: Because, normally, one of the purposes of the secretions and the odors is to attract men. In other species, we can see this very clearly—in the dog, when the bitch is in heat—

GUEST: Right.

DOCTOR: And many males are flocking around. . . .

GUEST: Yeah, right. Right. Well, I thought so, too, although one thought did cross my mind that, perhaps, from an anthropological point of view, this smell could become unpleasant to men who were maybe closet queens, due to the culture or whatever—that it was a biological number happening that would have controlled population, you know, if suddenly that odor became unpleasant to the men.

DOCTOR: Hey, you think that these a—

ENGINEER: Is that a weird theory!

DOCTOR: You think that these deodorant sprays are really, let's see here, are really tools of Planned Parenthood—right?

GUEST: Oh, yeah.

DOCTOR: Or Zero Population Growth.

GUEST: Yeah, they're the most horrible things! I wouldn't want any of my friends to drink any of that stuff; and that, y'know, just ruins the ecology of the—

DOCTOR: Well, you say—and I think it's true—that many

men say they're not interested in oral sex because they don't like the odor.

GUEST: Yeah. But I think if they just got down there and burrowed around for a while, they'd adapt—they'd get used to it. I know people that dig it, that no matter, some guys say the funkier the better, y'know, it's really real. You know, I believe in bathing and I know the hairs collect the smells and all that; you have to wash the hair very well.

DOCTOR: Incidentally, the definitive work on oral sex is called *Oragenitalism** by G. Legman, and it's about 360 pages explaining every conceivable variation, position—it even gets down so to speak, to the kind of lighting you should have in the room, the elevation of the bed and the furnishings in the room.

GUEST: How fantastic! And the guy's name is "Legman"?

DOCTOR: Legman—L-e-g-m-a-n. G. Legman believes that the function of pubic hair was to collect the secretions, because when man walked on all fours, of course, then the pubic hairs would collect the secretions and act as a sexual stimulant.

GUEST: Right, yeah.

DOCTOR: So, what do you recommend?

GUEST: Women should take a taste test of themselves every once in a while and eat a lot of yogurt.

DOCTOR: Why does that help?

GUEST: Well, I think yogurt has the same bacteria that should be present there in order for it to taste good. I've never tried putting yogurt in directly, but—

DOCTOR: A yogurt—yogurt douche?

GUEST: Yeah, I've never tried that but, you know, it might be something.

DOCTOR: It might be something.

GUEST: But I know that if I take yogurt—

DOCTOR: Plain or—

GUEST: I know I taste very—

* Now called *The Intimate Kiss*, Warner Paperback Library.

DOCTOR: Blueberry?

GUEST: No one's ever complained about my taste. No, straight, plain yogurt, none of that sugared stuff. Lay off that sugar. Healthy yogurt. Unpasteurized, if they can get it.

DOCTOR: What about the many women who are leery about participating in oral sex.

GUEST: Well, I must admit that eating pussy is easier than sucking cock.

DOCTOR: (turning to engineer) Well, that's, let's see—we can't—is that all right? (Background—someone says "It's all right.")

DOCTOR: You could've said "penis."

GUEST: Oh, penis, well—

DOCTOR: Well, so why is it easier? A lot of men complain that it's not easier because the clitoris is so small they have trouble finding it.

GUEST: Oh, well, they just—they have to look if they want to find out where it is, you know. A lot of 'em are afraid to look.

DOCTOR: You recommend strong light?

GUEST: No, but just enough to maybe see by—a little, teeny, tiny bit.

DOCTOR: What would you say to a woman who said, "Gee, I'd like to try that, but I just feel somehow there's something wrong with—"

GUEST: So demeaning and debasing and all. Well—

DOCTOR: "—there's something wrong with putting my mouth on a penis."

GUEST: It's ah—

DOCTOR: And this is reinforced, of course, by so many things. Like, in a way, the worst curse you could say, right, 's a ten-letter word that busted Lenny Bruce, right?

GUEST: Yeah, right, yeah. Ends in -e-r, right?

DOCTOR: Yeah, right. And it's not gonna bust us, okay? That's one of the worst things that you could call someone. I think because of that kind of attitude a lot of ladies are reluctant. Do you find that an unpleasant chore?

GUEST: No, not at all. I certainly did in the beginning, though, when I harbored some hostilities towards men. But I got to the point where I almost would—when I was hooking—I got to the point where I would rather suck a guy off than ball him. It was less intimate in a way, but more intimate from another aspect, you know. But, at least, it was away from his face, which is where most people communicate so it was really less personal. And probably I felt it was cleaner than his mouth. I didn't—some of my customers even drank and smoked and smelled foul, and tasted terrible.

DOCTOR: Yeah, cigarettes and alcohol really turn you off.

GUEST: That's really bad; yeah. But I got so I really liked it, and I like it still.

DOCTOR: Incidentally, I know, Margo, you met the guest we had last week—and she told us she had been a call girl for three months, and that wasn't a very long time, but you just mentioned that you had been a "hooker" and I was thinking earlier this week, I guess maybe we should have some kind of balance. I asked a lady I know, who is a suburban housewife, to appear on the show and she was very reluctant to do so.

GUEST: Well, I don't blame her; it may ruin her reputation.

DOCTOR: Aren't you worried about your reputation being ruined?

GUEST: Oh, no. It can only be enhanced.

DOCTOR: Umm. Ah, okay. This is KSAN-FM, San Francisco, and it's half a minute till 10:00. We're talking with Margo St. James and this is commercial time.

Commercial—Music Odyssey

FEMALE CALLER: I wanted to ask Margo what kind of exercises you can do so that you don't get tired when you're sucking your man off. Like, my mouth always gets tired.

GUEST: Hmm. Well, sometimes you can hardly avoid that

if he's got a big one, and if your mouth has to stay open too wide for a long period of time.

FEMALE CALLER: Yeah, well, do you know if there's anything to do? I have a fairly small mouth and it's, you know, it gives him pleasure and I like to do it, but I get very tired. Do you know if there's anything I could do for that?

GUEST: Well, you could practice on carrots or cucumbers, something like that, you know, to strengthen your mouth muscles.

DOCTOR: Well, if she ran, right, wouldn't she develop better breath control?

GUEST: Sure. Sure. Your breathing may have a lot to do with it. Maybe when—y'know sometimes when you're really doing a job you have a hard time getting air in there.

FEMALE CALLER: I have a question concerning vaginal infections and psychosomatic illness.

DOCTOR: Yes.

FEMALE CALLER: Where a woman's head is at can affect infections of that type. In other words, I have been having recurring bouts of trichomonas and they don't seem to be coming from anywhere and they disappear. And I am wondering if that is a reflection of where my head is at concerning myself sexually.

DOCTOR: It seems to be with a lot of women that they get vaginal infections if they are not feeling well. If their head's not in a good place, you know. If they are upset, often they will get a vaginal infection, even though the trichomonas [infection] is caused by a parasite. You can take some of the secretions and look at them under the microscope, and see these one-celled organisms moving quickly across the field of the microscope. But this is another of the diseases, and there are many like this, where, not only is a causative organism required, but also a decline in a person's general state of health, either mental or physical health.

FEMALE CALLER: What I am asking is, can the mental state

bring it on by itself? Or does there have to be some outside cause? In other words, perhaps it is not trichomonas, perhaps it is just the symptoms of trich psychologically induced.

DOCTOR: That could very well be, but usually the physician that examines you will take the secretions and examine them under a microscope. Each of these infections, like yeast infections and trichomonas, has a specific secretion, a specific odor which a lot of doctors can recognize, without even taking a microscope specimen.

FEMALE CALLER: Well, all the times I have had it treated, I have never had specimens taken.

DOCTOR: A competent gynecologist could tell just by the appearance and the odor. You might ask specifically to have a specimen taken next time you have this problem.

FEMALE CALLER: What I'm wondering now, though, is if I need a gynecologist or a psychiatrist. It's really getting to be a bummer—this is happening all the time. And it is very convenient for me to say, you know, well, I can't have sex because I have an infection.

DOCTOR: Well, all gynecologists practice psychiatry to some degree, and the very best gynecologists are also excellent psychiatrists.

FEMALE CALLER: Uh-huh. Oh well, at least now I know it is all in my head, but I'm not alone.

DOCTOR: It may not be all in your head. I am just suggesting that this may bring it on in some people, not in everyone. But it is very much involved, for many ladies do find that when they are upset they get more vaginal infections.

FEMALE CALLER: Uh-huh. Okay. Thank you very much.

DOCTOR: Okay. You're welcome. Margo, do you have any treatment for vaginal infections which plague a lot of ladies?

GUEST: I prefer to treat trich with—I get it once in a great while—with Flagyl suppositories and, if I keep a close watch, I will know right away if I come in contact with it, and I will up my yogurt intake. I don't douche normally, but I occasionally will douche with some Tide. Vinegar used to be the thing to neutralize the scene down there, but Tide seems to be the thing that washes everything; gets rid of the trich better than anything.

DOCTOR: Is that biodegradable?

GUEST: No. I don't know. Might be; now you know everybody is putting that on their box—

MALE CALLER: I phoned up to find out—Am I on the air?

DOCTOR: Yes, you're on the air.

MALE CALLER: Good—beautiful. What about venereal disease? Is there any way to know . . .

DOCTOR: You could ask, but some people aren't aware themselves. Usually people won't have sex when they know they have a venereal disease.

MALE CALLER: There's no rule of thumb to be able to—just dig on a certain part of the anatomy of another person?

DOCTOR: You mean to look, to make sure?

MALE CALLER: Exactly.

DOCTOR: If someone had a chancre, which is the first lesion of syphilis . . .

MALE CALLER: Right.

DOCTOR: He or she would have a painless, usually painless, sore or ulcer and it's usually around the genital areas. Usually it's on the penis, maybe on the shaft of the penis just below the glans. Or sometimes it may be on the glans; it may be on the lips of the vagina.

MALE CALLER: Uhh—uhh

DOCTOR: Let me just continue—

MALE CALLER: Aside from that—

DOCTOR:—Just hold on a minute, because I haven't finished yet and it's important, that's why I want to continue. They may also appear *anywhere* that sexual contact has been made, so if you have a break in the skin of your finger, for example, you might get a chancre on the finger. Or you might get it on the tongue, or on the roof of the mouth.

MALE CALLER: Does a chancre look any different than something we might normally have? Uhh—what you call a chancre to me a layman, I don't know a chancre. It's a lesion, right?

DOCTOR: Yeah. It's like—it's a sore. A canker sore, but a bigger canker sore.

MALE CALLER: Right.

DOCTOR: It doesn't hurt like a canker sore. It would sort of be that kind of sore, you know, the kind of thing that's open and sort of punched out. It has a rim—

MALE CALLER: Far out.

DOCTOR: That kind of thing. That's what you would look for.

MALE CALLER: That's the only way—but basically that's the only thing you have to think about or be concerned about. It's just something like that, in any kind of sexual encounter?

DOCTOR: Well, it's also possible to get other kinds of venereal diseases, such as gonorrhea, anyway sexual contact is made. But in the male, of course, there usually would be a discharge or pus from the penis.

MALE CALLER: Far out.

DOCTOR: In the female very often there are no symptoms, so it's hard to tell.

MALE CALLER: Far out. Well, I was just trying to figure out how to look at it without having to think of anything or to—you know—to consciously exert oneself to perform or to do something new and dangerous, supposedly. Morally speaking. To do something new and supposedly taboo. There are no taboos, except for, shall we say, health matters, right?

DOCTOR: Well, you know, taboos are in your own head. I mean, if you—

MALE CALLER: Yeah. But not really. You know—

DOCTOR: I didn't mean yours in particular—in one's own head. People's heads.

MALE CALLER: Uh-huh. Well, I hope not.

DOCTOR: Okay. Thanks for your call. Good night. Let's go

to another call. Good evening. You're on the air. This is Gene Schoenfeld. . . . We're going to play a little music now, while we adjust some technical difficulties.

MUSIC: "Rocket 69"—Todd Rhodes (Album: "Super Rock")

MALE CALLER: Listen, I'd like to ask you a question about —something you were talking about on the radio tonight. Eating out. I have a lady whose clitoris is particularly small—and I'd like to know—I'd like to ask Margo if there was a way of possibly increasing the size of a lady's clitoris by some kind of stimulation— I mean, you know, like—

GUEST: You mean—increasing it permanently, you mean.

MALE CALLER: Increasing the size of it—

GUEST: Well, the size increases with stimulation at the time.

MALE CALLER:—yes, it's true. Yes, but the clitoris itself is very small and I'd like to know if there is something I could do myself to work on, creating a different size of it.

GUEST: Well I—I've never found anything like that happening. It's like the story of a man—

MALE CALLER:—I mean eating it—even very large stimulation—it's—it still seems to be very small and I'd like to know if there's anything I could do to—

GUEST: It doesn't stand up by itself? When you play with it with your tongue?

MALE CALLER: Ahh, yes, it does, but it's very small. And I'd like—I'd, you know, really like to have it be larger. But—I'd like to know if you could tell me anything I could do—to do—

DOCTOR: Why would you like it larger?

MALE CALLER: Ahh—somewhat behind my complaint is having trouble of location—and somewhat behind her complaint is not having incre—uhh—very large-scale satisfaction behind it. I would feel that she would have larger satisfaction behind it—

GUEST:—If she had a larger clit—I just can't follow the logic in that at all. I think—more stimulation with the tongue, and maybe create a little vacuum when you're doing it to her with your mouth, you know—and over a little more area below the clit—with your tongue.

MALE CALLER: Right.

GUEST: Run it up and down—

MALE CALLER: You were saying this one about finger insertion.

GUEST: Yeah.

MALE CALLER: Ahhmm, do you think that would help?

GUEST: I think that—I think that—that helps quite a bit, but it widens the area of stimulation—it just—it's an additive to—

MALE CALLER: I'll tell you, the lady seems to be very stimulated behind what I'm doing, but I, you know, I really would like to increase the size of her stimulation. I mean for her pleasure, rather than mine. Ahh, this is like what we—like what's the name of the expression—ahh, Queen's position, right?

GUEST: Yeah.

MALE CALLER: And I was looking to increase her—her stimulation behind it.

GUEST: You say you already do the Queen's position.

MALE CALLER: Yes, I do that position.

GUEST: Well—ahmmm—it seems strange to me. It's like wishing my boyfriend had a bigger cock or something—if maybe he'd jack-off more it would grow. But, I see that I just—really, that's not true; there's nothing you can do. Perhaps—

MALE CALLER: Okay, okay—well I—

GUEST: There are operations where the labia—

MALE CALLER: Well, I mean it's just like—just like a dude who has a very small dick—

GUEST: Yeah?

MALE CALLER: You know—ahh, I guess that's—you know, I guess that's what's happening.

GUEST: Well, let me ask you this: are the labia oversized? And covering the clitoris?

MALE CALLER: Ah, no. It's pretty much very open.

GUEST: Oh well, that sounds all right to me. I don't think there's anything you could do about enlarging it—you have what you get when you're born, I think. That's about it.

DOCTOR: I don't think there's any relationship between that and feelings, or the ability to receive or give pleasure.

GUEST: It's in your head, man.

MALE CALLER: Yes, indeed.

DOCTOR: Right, that's—it's in your head. That's the answer.

MALE CALLER: Okay, okay. Thank you very much.

DOCTOR: You're very welcome.

MALE CALLER: Good night.

DOCTOR: Good night.

Commercial—Grisedick Malt Liquor (pronounced Grees-a-Dick)

FEMALE CALLER: I want to speak to Margo please.

DOCTOR: All right, Margo.

GUEST: Yes?

FEMALE CALLER: I have a problem. I guess someone else had the same problem too. But I have never experienced an orgasm and I was wondering if there is something that can be done and at this point I am wondering if it is psychological or physical or what.

GUEST: Well, do you play with yourself at all?

FEMALE CALLER: No, I never have.

GUEST: Well, I think that would be a good place to start. By yourself, perhaps in front of a mirror and tell yourself how beautiful you are. Do it for God or whatever. In the *Whole Earth Catalog* there's a little booklet you can send for for 35 cents, quite extensive, on knowing one's body. It has excellent diagrams and pictures of the anatomy. You can even use a vibrator, if you—

FEMALE CALLER: Yeh, I was thinking of that too.

GUEST: Yeh.

DOCTOR: A lot of gynecologists recommend using a vibrator for women who have never had an orgasm to teach them what an orgasm feels like.

GUEST: Good luck.

FEMALE CALLER: Yeh.

GUEST: Yeh, let me know.

DOCTOR: That is one of the most common problems of ladies. It is one of the most common letters I get. Women who have difficulty achieving orgasm—and I guess most or all women have this problem sometime in their lives.

GUEST: Well, I didn't find out about things like that until twenty-two.

DOCTOR: How did you find out?

GUEST: I read Kinsey.

DOCTOR: Okay, thanks for your call. Good night.

FEMALE CALLER: Hello, Doctor Schoenfeld?

DOCTOR: Yes, this is Doctor Schoenfeld.

FEMALE CALLER: I wanted to speak toward the subject of Tantric Yoga that you mentioned earlier in the program.

DOCTOR: We touched on the subject before. What did you want to say about Tantric Yoga?

FEMALE CALLER: I would like for you to carry on some dialogue between the two of you regarding that subject. Part of Tantric seems to be that genital union is the high experience of that type of Yoga.

DOCTOR: Well, it is curious, isn't it, that there are various kinds of yogas and in some sex is prohibited or discouraged. But in Tantric yoga the sexual act is paramount, primarily the woman facing the male, sitting on his lap—

GUEST: Yab-yum is probably the most popular position.

DOCTOR:—With her legs around his buttocks, penetration is maintained. In this position the penis can stay within the vagina even though the male doesn't have an erection. And it's said that if the Yab-yum position is maintained for a period of two or three hours, then there is a state which has been described as that of a third kind of existence—the male and the female merge and there is a third being.

GUEST: A oneness.

DOCTOR: A oneness, a togetherness.

GUEST: One of the things that happens in the beginning, and during the achieving of this, is breathing together. And it is not one person leading the breathing or anything like that. It just begins to happen with both people breathing exactly the same.

FEMALE CALLER: In connection with the exercises that you were speaking of earlier, the vaginal exercises. Would this not be in relation here?

GUEST: Yes.

DOCTOR: Oh, yes, this would be especially important in Yab-yum.

GUEST: Right.

DOCTOR: Do you have any other questions?

FEMALE CALLER: Thank you.

DOCTOR: We have time for one more fast call and then we are going to have—

(According to producer Rona Elliot this is the end of the program and there were no more calls.)

Index